Brain [

THEIR STORIES, MY JOURNEY

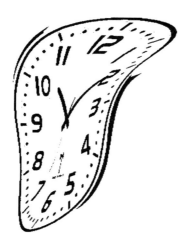

LYDIA WINSLOW

BRIGHTON PUBLISHING LLC
435 N. HARRIS DRIVE
MESA, AZ 85203

Brain Damaged
Their Stories, My Journey

Lydia Winslow

Brighton Publishing LLC
435 N. Harris Drive
Mesa, AZ 85203
www.BrightonPublishing.com

Copyright © 2013

ISBN 13: 978-1-62183-123-5
ISBN 10: 1-62183-123-X

Printed in the United States of America

First Edition

Cover Design: Tom Rodriguez

DEDICATION

This book is dedicated to my brain damaged friends, and those others who love me the way I need to be loved.

ACKNOWLEDGEMENTS

Thank you to my amazing husband, Skip, for just being. Thanks to my son, Ian, who awes me more each day. You are the man I prayed you would be and much more.

Thanks to Dorothy Casper for unconditional love and respect.

Thank you, Peggy-pig, for teaching me to understand.

Thank you to my sister, Irene, who understands why I had to bring up the bad stuff.

Thanks to my colleagues, and all at Brighton Publishing who read, improved, added, subtracted, and clarified.

FOREWORD

F ixing brain damaged patients is not in the job description of a Theatre Major.

My career path began on stage as an off-Broadway actor, moved off stage as I became a lighting technician on Broadway for *Jesus Christ Superstar*, off Broadway as a member of the innovative and celebrated LaMaMa Troupe, and then off-off Broadway editing and marketing books. Before entering the profession of speech pathology, I worked for MCA Records writing public relations pamphlets for the label's country music division as well as liner notes and information on the back of album jackets.

Following that, I edited advance material for *The New York Times Book List*. Throughout various career roles and job opportunities, I have continuously written, edited and published civic newsletters. I've had my nonfiction works published in two internationally recognized hobby periodicals: *Garden Railways Magazine* and *AW NUTS Magazine*.

A chance viewing of a TV show, Dr. Kildare, in 1963 in which Harry Guardino played an aphasic, was the pebble that redirected the flow of my life's work. The actor's poignant portrayal of a stroke victim who was unable to speak still haunts me.

In my twenties, when I first started my practice in speech-language pathology (SLP), I was insensitive, self-absorbed and ignorant. I had graduated from New York University with an aptly named B.S. degree in drama, and then from the City University of New York with a more useful Master of Arts in Speech Pathology. Before returning to university five years later for my masters, I had high ambitions of becoming the quintessential lighting designer on Broadway. It is a very narrow scope of ambition in view of the professionals who monopolized the industry in a very finite place: New York City.

I adopted the view that New Yorkers have, that Manhattan is the center of the universe. After my training as a speech pathologist, I assumed I had cache in my new profession as I had gotten my educational credentials there and then landed a plum of a student externship at the Manhattan VA Hospital. Topping off a perfect resume, I went on to a position at a prestigious rehabilitation center in Westchester County, just north of New York City. I was leading a charmed life, but I knew nothing and did not know enough to admit it. My poor patients! They had gone to an expert in a field expecting that expert to know what she was doing. I was winging it and my early patients no doubt suffered from my lack of know-how and experience.

Forty years later, I've accumulated much valuable and some exotic knowledge practicing what I call "Extreme Medicine" in state psychiatric hospitals, in group home communities for those who have multiple handicaps, in prisons, and in long-term acute care hospitals in widely divergent populations.

What began as a couple pieces of writing about some of my quirky patients became mini-portraits of people whose lives were at the tipping point. Through the writing of these portraits I saw therein my own journey of integration of myself both professionally and personally. I have uncovered in myself a capacity for patience and a depth of attachment to such a variety of people I never would have gravitated toward had the meetings with these folks been merely social.

Through the years, with every new introduction to patients who did not plan to end up in an intensive care unit desperately ill, new questions arose: *Could this happen to me? How would I handle being helpless? Does anyone leave home planning to never again return? Can I imagine myself ending, not in death but forever changed?*

The people mentioned here have been forever changed. Some did return home, but they have been constitutionally altered. Befriending each of them has constitutionally altered me, too. As a medical speech pathologist, I have treated scores of people in their days following brain damage.

I have had a front row seat to the long, tedious, and painful process of recovery for those I have met, cared for, and come to love during my forty years in practice.

"Don't stare at that person," is something parents warn their kids. Whether through recent accident or from birth, physical and mental impairments draw stares and pity or worse—avoidance. Whether one says, "There but for the grace of God go I," or "just bad karma," or "wrong place, wrong time," we don't want to *be* that impaired person; we don't want to *know* that person.

Sitting around for many years with colleagues telling war stories about the antics of our patients, I realized that you can't make this stuff up. When I put pen to paper to make good on my promise to log the strange people and events, I realized the value of the relationships I made with my patients, and what they meant to me. Then I saw that it was also about what I meant to them, how they thanked me. I have, in writing this book, discovered the reason for putting years into working with broken people.

From my present perspective after nearly four decades in this career, I see that I was looking for my own definition. Not just in a career but as a person. I began with a job designing Broadway lights that would enhance actors, while I remained invisible myself. Then I intimately inserted myself into the lives of folks at their most fragile moments. Still remaining invisible, I realize now that I was spotlighting my patients in their recovery.

FROM MY PERSPECTIVE

I don't for a moment believe that my parents nurtured my self-esteem. I feel both of them in their own ways damaged my self-worth. My mother constantly compared me to other little girls, wishing she could shape me into a well-behaved doll. She held my chin between her thumb and index finger and crooned, "A face only a mother could love."

Here is how I saw it:

I recognized my father as a brilliant man who made some lousy choices. Still, my father criticized the choices I made in friends and in school—that is, when he paid attention to me at all. I suppose I felt I deserved their criticism, his neglect, and their behavior toward me. Along with a legacy of rotten self-esteem, my family bequeathed me a lack of respect for authority. I consider that, perhaps, I did not know the rules or didn't choose to play by the rules. I am congenitally tactless.

I am also the child of a community of alcoholics. It was much like trying to balance on a surfboard in a wild unpredictable ocean. As James Joyce may have put it, "I had a farther and a smother for parents." I felt that my dad couldn't care less, and I thought that my mother was trying to work through her own dysfunction by giving me enemas when I didn't poop once a day, dressing her tomboy up in frilly, ruffled dresses, and showing me off as the product of her late-in-life, trophy-wife marriage. Before this, her second marriage, she had spent fifteen childless years as a young widow; she was used to doing as she pleased. And she was controlling. When I chose to make my own decisions, she slammed me around. Bouncing me across the room was her idea of nurturing.

I had protective quirks such as stopping up my ears or pushing on my closed eyes until I saw pinpoints of light like a starry night. I think I did these things so I wouldn't have to hear or see the arguments that turned into bloody brawls or experience dear Dad puking his hangover away on the other side of the wall, or finding his car in the middle of the lawn at dawn.

I suppose my most vulnerable age was five. At five I was hospitalized twice: once for tonsil and adenoid removal (a rite of passage for early boomers), and then for a painful appendix. Five was around the time that my mother was hospitalized for several weeks for some sort of liver problem. Five was the age when I broke my nose. My mother blamed me for tripping over a toy xylophone. She never took me to have it treated or repaired. It doesn't take a whole lot to bring me back to being five years old. A mean look, a rejection from a friend or lover, a challenge to an accomplishment and I feel five years old, again and again and again.

Cruel playmates teased me about my father. "Your father's a drunk!" they taunted. I tried to deny it, was reluctant to face this fact. By day, my father was a busy, successful businessman. When my dad drank, the change in him scared me. I didn't like the metamorphosis from the articulate, witty, companionable daddy that once danced with his little girl and sometimes helped her with her schoolwork, to the disheveled, smelly man who fell into his recliner after weaving his car home from the bar.

My father and a group of businessmen started Rova Farms, a Russian enclave. The name comes from initials translated from Cyrillic: R.O.O.V.A. and it stands for Russian Consolidated Mutual Aid Society. When he and I were together at Rova Farms and it was time for us to go home, friends' parents would often intervene. They insisted, "Jack, you go on. We will take the child. She can't go with you." Afraid for his safety, I insisted that we follow him, and I watched through the car's windshield as his car on the road ahead weaved caroming from shoulder-to-shoulder of the two-lane to our house. In present day dream-mares I watch, terror-filled for my father.

My mother seemed helpless in dealing with the husband who was the drunk. I don't know how much she had invested in him at that point in their lives. I don't know how much she had helped. Instead she turned to her prepubescent daughter and gave me a *mandate*: "He loves you, go sit on his lap. Tell him to stop drinking. Fix him." Shrinking away from the very thought, I begged her, "I can't. He smells. I'm scared. I can't. I just can't."

When I was twelve, my father was told that he had cancer. He refused to accept this and traveled to the major cities around us—Philadelphia, Baltimore, New York—for a solution, for a cure. This prideful man who made his life out of courting people, out of building associations, out of running companies and organizations, this man would not allow doctors to remove his larynx, his ability to verbalize. He searched for other fixes, and ultimately took too long. The cancer had insidiously taken his larynx, his esophagus and then his lungs. He continued to drink, and I thought he was totally unbearable to be around. His misery was everybody's misery. He poisoned my life and I wished him dead. I said it out loud and said it often. I prayed for it. Please just *die*. And then he did. And my fifteen-year-old brain created a superstition, an unhealthy association between two disparate events: I wished him dead and he died; therefore, I killed him. In a twisted way, I fulfilled my mother's mandate to me. I fixed him good.

I felt that I surely was a headache for both of my parents. Today there are labels for the kind of kid I was. But back then I was just *bad*. When I was in kindergarten, the principal caught me peeing on the hallway floor. I recall thinking, *Why go to the trouble of opening the bathroom door, then the stall door, and then lifting my skirt, and then finally pulling down my panties? Might as well just pee in the hall.* But then the principal discovered me. In mid-pee. I felt bad. Don't know the label for the emotion I was feeling. Guilt perhaps. Shame perhaps. Guilt and shame were my lifelong companions.

Other questionable hobbies I engaged in, for whatever reason, were: pulling chairs out from under a classmate just as she was sitting, and piling as many books as I could hold, and then smashing the lot on someone's head. In my elementary school I caused as much havoc as I could. Reader, while these memories may elude me now, the reminders of my lousy behavior are immortalized in each and every report card. I saved them all.

I was no better at home. A bright, sunny day may find me sitting, enjoying the warm breeze, on the shoulder of our rural road. I sat waiting for any car to crest the hill with no opportunity to evade the board I put in its path. My board had three-inch nails sticking out of it. It was a science experiment. I wanted to see if the car would go airborne when the tires blew. *Would the driver be injured?* Bonus.

I managed to find bad company with whom to associate. Were these delinquents the bad influence? Or was I? Anyway, put two iffy kids with twisted fantasies together and you have a dangerous situation. My friend Millie and I challenged ourselves in the off-season of the resort we lived in. Who could break into an empty vacation house the quickest? I was midway into box-knifing a window screen when I got busted. The groundskeeper grabbed me, and dragged me crying to my parents who he knew to be in the bar. My mother was scandalized—not *her* daughter. I don't remember being punished. I know I deserved to be—wanted to be—for I had done wrong. Either that or I could not back then distinguish "punished" from "parenting."

My coup de grace when I was oh, about ten years old, was destroying the vacant summer camp dorm. Once more, I don't recall a deliberateness as in, "I'm going to do this because." I just did it. I ripped mattresses, broke windows, toppled bunks, threw garbage. Oh yeah, I had a ball. Once again, not punished. Word around the resort was that "someone" thrashed the camp. *I wonder who?*

Another year (I was now fourteen), yet another delinquent girlfriend: I visited Linda and her family in Queens for a weekend. We were bored. We were restless. We connived. She said the neighbors were away on a cruise and left her parents in charge of their house. We broke in, or had a key, whatever, found their car keys and opened the garage. There it was, their car just sitting there. We hit an early snag. Neither of us could drive a stick. I had tried once the previous year when I decided to drive my mother's car to a friend's house because I was just too lazy to walk. This unsuccessful experience qualified me to be the designated driver. I managed to start the neighbor's car's engine and I even knew how to step on the clutch to shift. I threw that car into reverse so fast we plowed into the brick wall of Linda's neighbor's house. The car stalled, stuck backend into trouble. Not punished. Linda was a glib liar, "We saw these two guys in the car, then heard a crash!"

Destruction of property wasn't the only thing I engaged in. Cruel words came flying out of my mouth wounding those who dared to befriend me. I didn't mean to hurt. As soon as the barbs were flung, I felt remorse. I lost a few friends but kept many more. The ones that stuck around didn't punish either. Unless you count loving me as a sort of punishment. I knew I didn't deserve their loyalty. How did I come to deserve their love?

Throughout my childhood and teen years, I protected myself by hurting others before they hurt me. I couldn't let others discover what I knew: that inside of me was wormy with the stench of rot, of writhing acid, of *rage*. My principal, my parents, and later my bosses didn't need to punish me for being bad—I actively and frequently punished myself. The "me" that was visible to classmates and other acquaintances was tall, red-haired, unsmiling, sarcastic and nasty. Like a timid, small prey animal fleetingly glimpsed in the forest clearing, my vulnerability was seen only by those whom I allowed close to me. I thought—and still think—it's cruel that the body I was assigned didn't reveal the vulnerable personality within.

My father's death when I was fifteen left me abandoned with unresolved business. I was angry beyond words for him dying when I'd wished him to. That's too much responsibility and power for one young girl. He wasn't there when I was trying to establish myself as an individual. The angst of those hormonal teenaged formative years combined with his death left me with my identity incomplete. And a lot of rage.

I dragged this burden of rage around for years, like the festering albatross around the fisherman's neck I read about in my English lit class. Disrupting and destroying and verbally maiming didn't get the response I needed: an understanding heart. I took another direction: I overcompensated. I did more, I learned more. I set out to show I was worthy of closeness and respect. Overcompensating didn't get the response I needed either. I was clueless. I was lost. Group and individual therapies eventually let me see that I needed to purge the rage and forgive myself for whatever I was guilty of.

Ultimately, I chose to intimately work with people who are very sick. I study them. Maybe if these very sick people could be fixed, so could I. And if I had a hand in fixing them, I'd feel good about myself. I needed to feel good about myself. I needed to impress others. I needed to challenge myself by being skilled, learning more, doing the best. By being the best, I would be bulletproof. I'd guarantee a job and respect. I didn't know that by trying so hard that I would alienate the people I worked with. I should have.

So why did I go into the "healing arts"?

I fix people. I'm good at it. I approach my work with pride and consider myself a tireless, productive worker. Yet my bosses or co-workers have seldom complimented me. But my patients have been very generous in their thanks, and I absolutely have dedicated myself to them.

I have gained a reputation for being my patients' strongest advocate. One supervisor pointed out to me that sometimes advocating for your patient can be contrary to the wishes of the doctor or the health care provider. My stroke victim might benefit from two more weeks as an inpatient, and then go to a decent rehabilitation center. The insurance provider has decided not to cover rehabilitation and wants them discharged now. The doctor concurs and writes the order. Lydia objects, assertively approaches the doctor and the case manager, and gives reasons why the patient should not go yet. A glance between the doctor and the case manager tells Lydia: oops you're out of bounds, again.

I know I have a responsibility to the facility and to the people with whom I work. The fact that I care for my patients is clear, that's why I chose this profession. The people I need to support and nurture are the people who care for my patients alongside me. Despite that I am a member of a medical team I have, at times, considered the people I worked next to and alongside of my competition, but for what? For my patients' love? My bosses' respect? My *father's* respect? Recognition of self-worth and a job well done? I have seldom gotten praise for a job well done. But I have always gotten appreciation from my patients and their families.

Maybe I should have received more guidance, more constructive criticism early on. In hindsight, it was not to my advantage to be hired at prestigious facilities: the VA, the Westchester rehab center. Rather than humbly absorbing all the experience I could have from my mentors, I isolated myself in a cocoon of arrogance. Had I exposed my vulnerability, I would have received more support and guidance. I wouldn't have placed myself in situations in which I alienated others. I would love to have a do-over.

I thought I should work hard, work long, show ambition, and be productive. My work ethic often times brought me my supervisors' coldness and co-workers' suspicion. Did I make others look bad because their numbers did not meet my standards? Was I too smart? Or was it I who radiated competitiveness? Maybe I was looking for love in all the wrong places. Love from a pitiable human with a hand out for help when they are down and out? Of course they "loved" me. Did I go into the service profession because I was guaranteed of this love? Why does anyone become a therapist? Is it really selfless?

Am I minimizing my attachment to my coworkers and bosses? I

remain close to many of my colleagues. Am I putting too much emphasis on the attachment to my patients? I am trying to understand why in over forty years of working as a speech-language pathologist, my greatest reward is my lasting friendship with some, my memory of others, and a number of keepsakes that evoke memories of still others. The respect and love I continue to search for should have come from my father. My everlasting heartbreak is that I never really knew him. He and I have much unfinished business. I've spent my life trying to find the "me" that was never really defined. I feel like a jigsaw puzzle with pieces missing: you do what you can with what you have, but the whole never really satisfies. I'll try to be better, Daddy, I'll be good.

My scribblings over the last ten years have become this book about meeting—and then loving—my brain damaged patients, and as a bonus, getting to know and love myself. I also have grown through the gifts each patient has lovingly and unselfishly given to me.

I sit now with my glass of wine in my sunroom looking over my beautiful piece of South Carolina property and reflect upon how far I have come geographically and personally. I have accumulated respect for myself and have grown to like the person I've become.

I take a little from each person I treat and pass it along. My patients have been excellent tutors.

A NOTE ON CLOCK DRAWING

A clock begins many sections of this book. Clocks are familiar; we see them frequently throughout the day. We know that a clock is divided into twelve hours, which are duplicated for days and nights to denote twenty-four hours. We have functionally learned how to read a clock, to tell time by seeing the position of its two or three hands. Most of us are also adept at digital time but that's not what will be noted here. Because a clock is so much a part of one's life, it is a valuable tool in assessing neurological impairment.

The clocks in this book are the actual clocks drawn by my patients.

Those working with the brain-injured use clock drawing to evaluate dementia or delirium. I have always used clocks with my language-impaired patients. Language impairment occasionally comes along with or sometimes masks a cognitive impairment such as dementia. The clock gives clues as to the presence, character, and extent of a patient's impairment, including perception and use of space, ordering and sequence, symbolic use of numbers, attention to task, ability to follow aural or written directions, and the ability to draw.

The clocks reflect disability and the clocks tell time. Draw a line. This is your life line. Mark it at the age you are now. On one side your past, on the other your future. This line is a clock, too.

Lydia Winslow

PART ONE

LOOKING FOR ME

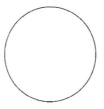

Anna

Glistening, near-naked bodies, impossibly perfect, strut along Ocean Drive, sneaking sidelong glances at those seated at very hip, sidewalk cafes. At eight in the evening, still hours before the club scene swings into action, the beautiful people pick through stone crabs, piling shells into pyramids. Looking across this pile of shells, it's difficult to imagine 1976 before the club scene, before the endless, tanned parade of young models, before the 1980 Mariel boatlift, which, in one fell swoop moved the middle class Jews out and the poor Cubans into Miami Beach's South Beach.

I had just arrived in South Florida from New York City. I was still in my twenties and I was a shiny-new speech-language pathologist. I was lucky enough to snatch a job working as a contract therapist for a practice on Lincoln Road in Miami Beach. My patients were mostly confined to their homes, and had recently been discharged from the hospital. My home health agency information sheet said that my patient, Anna H. was seventy-six and was in good health, except for a stroke, which affected her ability to communicate.

The address was a small building similar to others that lined the streets on that southern part of the island of Miami Beach, on the tip of South Beach. What was old is now new. And oh-so-hip. Her small apartment in a modest two story, pale-pink art deco building, opened right onto the beach. The building was no taller than two stories and was divided into four average-sized apartments. Each apartment had one bedroom, bath, a kitchen area with a back door and an entrance into the

1

living area through a screened in front porch. What was outstanding about this nondescript building was that it had occupied the very last lot on Ocean Drive, south of Biscayne Street, or what is now South Pointe Park, overlooking not only the ocean but Government Cut—the sea lane ocean liners use to access the Atlantic.

Three acres of palm stretched between Anna's building and the water, and Australian pine-dotted sandy dunes where, I later learned, Anna liked to walk. Across from this property was Fisher's Island—then relatively deserted—but now home to millionaires the likes of Oprah. This was 1976 and Miami Beach was very white, very Jewish, and very old. Anna's South Beach was a very poor area populated by the elderly on small, fixed incomes and by cocaine cowboy criminals immortalized on the popular 1980s TV series, *Miami Vice*. In those days the draw was the local favorite (and now world-famous) Joe's Stone Crabs, kitty-corner across the four-lane street from Anna's little home. Other than Joe's, tourists had no reason to venture into that residential area. But I had other business in that particular neighborhood. Sharing an alley with Joe's Stone Crabs was a nursing home called Four Freedoms, and not a half-block away another aptly named Hebrew Home for the Aged.

I worked at both of these facilities as a speech pathologist. I was young, fresh and optimistic. I couldn't imagine a future in which I would be any different except more successful—whatever that meant. Years later, after that area was nicknamed South Beach, I returned to Four Freedoms as a supervisor of rehab services, and as South Miami Beach morphed into SoBe, Four Freedoms was renamed South Point Rehab. Staffed then with young, pierced, pink-haired trendy therapists, the nursing home still housed sick, white, old people although now the majority of the staff and the patients were Cuban. As Miami Beach changed, so did I. And I had yet to even imagine the road I would travel.

I knocked on the door at Anna's beachside fourplex. No one answered. I tried the door to find it unlocked. I walked around to the back and spotted her. My lasting image of Anna was of her silhouetted against the early-morning sun, standing barefoot on the sand, looking out over the turquoise Atlantic, shielding her eyes with one wrinkled hand against the sun exploding the sea with diamonds. The breeze was blowing her blue cardigan sweater gently and her gray hair skimmed across her face and behind her. I imagined her as a fisherman's wife waiting for her husband or trying to spot the tall sailing ship that would bring back her pirate lover.

She saw me a moment later and walked over, smiling to greet me. She left her door unlocked, for there was nothing to protect inside: her belongings were modest, and there was nothing worth stealing. Subsequently, when I visited her, I just let myself in and waited for her. I don't know what she thought about out there on the sand; she never told me. She couldn't tell me because she had few words. The stroke took them away.

Anna was lean, almost sinewy, and tall, or it seems so in my mind's eye, and preferred shirtwaist dresses in the style of June Cleaver or Harriet Nelson. Her features were chiseled but soft like the smooth surfaces of rock sanded by time. I took her to be German, perhaps, European descended for sure. And she was South Beach tan.

Her home was modestly furnished: a small dining table and two chairs, and a simply furnished living area that welcomed whomever entered through her front porch. I entered and took one of the aluminum chairs at the table. The little house was clean with few personal touches. The furnishings were so generic that I wondered if Anna had rented the place furnished. She sat in the only other chair. If I was impressed one way or another by her, so far, I can't recall. I guess her greeting was appropriate. Certainly she was an unusual patient in that she walked without help and lived alone with no apparent care from another. When you've treated a number of catastrophically bitten people who were bed-bound and barely aware of you, a walking, talking person was a treat.

I returned Anna's steady gaze and introduced myself, told her why her doctor had sent me, and what I was there to do. Her gaze did not waver but she had yet to respond. I had nothing to do but begin the testing. I always started my language testing with easy commands from a generic standardized test: open your mouth, hold up your hand—that kind of thing. I'd then move on to questions that can be answered with a "yes" or "no." Following the questions, I had my patient point to something I would name, and then go on to short simple stories followed by questions about each story.

Anna had difficulty with everything I had asked her to do so far. She crinkled her forehead at the commands and only answered a few correctly. Her "yes's" and "no's" were not reliable. Although she listened with intensity, she could not recall facts from a paragraph she heard. I wanted to see if her inability to follow commands involved something physical, or a break in the signal from the intention center in her brain to her body, so I asked her to imitate what I did. She caught on well and followed my lead. Anna had some damage to the comprehension center of the brain due to her stroke.

What else was amiss? I wondered.

Taking control of her possible responses, I posed completion tasks such as "boy and…" trailing off and gesturing that she should finish the phrase. She performed fairly well. Her speech gave no indication of muscle weakness of the mouth or throat.

When I eased back on my control and began sentences left undone that my patient had to complete (such as "Last Sunday…") with the same inviting gesture to complete what was started, Anna strung together words which had recognizable structure but no meaning. Something on the order of, "Last Sunday…if you went out to the and bring back my house." Remembering my graduate school lessons from a mere three years ago, I knew that Anna presented me with a type of language disorder adversely affecting comprehension. I later came up with the label, "Wernicke's Aphasia" to describe this condition.

Adult "aphasia" means a loss or impairment of language following brain damage.

I also remembered that hallmarks of Wernicke's Aphasia, also referred to as sensory aphasia, included: words spoken smoothly but not with any meaningful substance, problems retrieving words, poor comprehension, and difficulty repeating. Sensory aphasics don't seem to know they are not communicating well. They have poor self-monitoring—they don't understand their own speech.

I used the rest of my test time to explore Anna's writing, reading, gesturing, and verbal expression. Our conversations were not typical. I would talk, she would listen and respond with actions and "not-words"—and I somehow understood. Or maybe I filled in blanks. Maybe I got it all wrong, I'll never know. Very basically, Anna did not understand much that was said to her. Although her speech had familiar rhythms, her verbal expression did not make sense. I set about to plan a course of action to improve Anna's communication. I left her with a business card and told her I would be back the next day.

As the screen door slapped shut behind me that first time, I thought about the prospect of living alone with an inability to adequately communicate.

We take so much for granted, I thought as I walked away.

All the times I visited Anna, she was alone. When I got to know her better, I took liberties. As she stared out over her ocean, I came inside and ferreted for clues as to whom I could call about her to get information, some background, in case something happened to her. I felt I had the right since I was referred to her by her primary physician and had a responsibility for her well-being. I just assumed that everyone had someone.

She had no address book. No pictures decorated the apartment walls that gave up hints of antecedents or bouncing grandchildren. Some of the usual detritus of day-to-day was scattered around: bank statements, newspapers, junk mail that waited to be tossed. But no hint of people.

In the beginning, I put my therapy books down on her kitchen table, waited for her to sit with me and started with our sessions. A certain personal protocol grew from visiting minimally verbal or nonverbal people in their homes. I had a routine. They knew why I was there. I told them my name, what they were to expect from me, and tenderly explored how much of what I said was understood, wholly or in part. I wrote down a lot of what I said aloud. It helped sometimes. If family members were present, it was easier. I could speak to the loved one with frequent glances at my patient knowing my message would be repeated to her once I left. With Anna, I was on my own.

She apparently had no family. Nor any friends. No one was ever there the same time as I was. How was I supposed to help her? I showed her pictures and asked her to repeat the names of the pictured items. I was somewhat successful in getting this tolerant woman to give back a recognizable word or two. I suppose I was quite proud of myself for being her crusader—the glamorous champion of communication who was going to restore life itself to this wordless woman. Not quite.

I supposed a neighbor took pity and time and stocked her refrigerator because she had food and she did not appear hungry or malnourished. I just supposed. She caught me furtively glancing into the refrigerator one day and just smiled. My curiosity aroused, I asked her frankly with words and gestures who had bought the groceries for her. She stood up, picked up her sweater then her purse. She walked out the door. I guessed I was to follow.

Anna lived in an area that would be desirable years later. In

Anna's time, the neighborhood was low-rise and poor. The apartments were filled with the elderly who overflowed their stoops onto the streets and beaches. Joe's Stone Crab, nearby, served the wannabe famous who waited for hours to be seated after subtly palming the maitre d' a large bill or two for the privilege of just being there.

I walked briskly to keep up with Anna, who knew just where she was going. She turned to me before entering a tiny Cuban grocery store—the kind that sells the incidentals one forgot when they went to the supermarket. For an instant I felt stupid. I assumed Anna to be European but thought that she must be Hispanic and that was why she can't understand my English. I usually explored a bit to see of my patients were more comfortable in another language but Anna seemed so…continental. Somehow, it didn't occur to me she might be Latin.

My poised erect-postured patient nodded her hello to the cashier and strolled down aisles, selecting items everyone needs: toilet paper, soup, coffee, cold cuts, the usual. She took longer to carefully select her fruits and a few vegetables. Wordlessly, she approached the cashier with me silently in tow. This was clearly her shopping trip—not ours. She handed the cashier a twenty-dollar bill, which apparently was sufficient, for she received change. Anna accepted her change silently, with a wry smile and a little shrug and threw it in her purse. The cashier displayed recognition of Anna, and Anna of the clerk, but neither spoke. Off we went back to her home.

I was dumbstruck. This was a woman who was neurologically impaired, who, because of her stroke, lost every vestige of verbal language. Yet, she maintained cognition, strategy, appreciation of options, humor, irony. She used a Cuban grocery not because she was Cuban but because she knew that the Cubans, still in a small minority on South Beach, would not presume to speak to her, an Anglo, in English. She did not have to speak to them. It was brilliant.

After the Cuban grocery-shopping trip, I accompanied Anna to many places one needs in order to maintain independence. My car came in handy as well, although she never complained when she had to walk many blocks to get places. She had a solid, apparently long-standing relationship with her bank. Instead of the teller's window, she chose a woman who sat at one of those desks in the lobby. I asked the bank woman if she was a personal banker.

She laughingly said, "No, but I help Mrs. H out when she comes

6

in. I recognize her from before her stroke. Anything I can do to make it easier for her, poor thing." It took me awhile to figure out that Anna had no concept left of the value of her money. Coins were confusing and so was the green money. To use a coin laundry, she took out all of her coins and just pushed them into the slot one by one until something fit. She used that coin as a model to choose others until she deposited enough to do her wash. She was clever.

I recalled the cashier at the grocery. Anna gave her a twenty although she had some smaller bills in her wallet. It made it easier to get change rather than choose the right amount of change to give the cashier. Now, in the bank, Anna's "personal banker," cashed her social security checks and changed her small bills, giving her twenties and fifties so she could continue shopping and laundering independently.

For many years since meeting Anna, I've often marveled at how resilient some people are, how thoughtful and clever they can be. Anna gave me a huge gift: the ability to interact with individuals on their own terms. I came to realize the wholeness of a person, and who they were before I came along. Treating Anna was exciting for the lessons she taught me. Much more excitement was yet in my future. Anna's independence meant more to her than the security of a boarding house. She was determined to live and die in her own home.

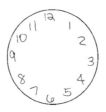

The Early Years: 1973-1975

Three years before Anna, after one year of coursework, I met my very first clients at the City College of New York speech clinic. After the course study, young therapists-to-be continue the learning process through hands-on work with flesh-and-blood, unsuspecting, speech impaired, humans.

In class, we went over the developmental stages of language acquisition. We were exposed to endless tables and appendices in textbooks. We learned the anatomy related to speaking and hearing. In my diagnostics course, I recall one assignment was to create an articulation test. We collected pictures from magazines that represented the sounds that words started with or ended with. Even back then in the 70s, I remember thinking, *Why are we doing this? Isn't there already a decent test instrument?*

What I definitely don't recall—in any of the coursework I sat through—was any instruction in how to engage young children in order to build rapport before evaluating their speech or language. Recently I glanced through a PowerPoint presentation on early childhood communication. I found a treasure trove of directions, suggestions, and resources appropriate for a speech therapist to use to access a young child's communication skills. Included were not only pointers on articulation, but also what to look for pragmatically: attention, interaction, parallel play, turn taking, and so on. But this PowerPoint was not yet available when I returned to the university in 1973 to learn my new trade.

In the university clinic, I was assigned a two-year-old to evaluate, and two victims, or rather *clients*, to treat: a ten-year-old who was labeled a schizophrenic and who didn't acknowledge me, and a young-adult stutterer for whom I was the seventh or eighth assigned therapist and who probably—no definitely—knew more than I did.

The two-year-old scared me the most. As an only child with no babysitting experience, I was at a total loss of how to start. My supervisor watched me from behind a two-way mirror, grading me on what I had learned so far. (Nothing.)

"Hi. My name is Miss Winslow—what's yours?" I sat on a chair, and then moved to the floor in order to sit and watch this tiny person who was oblivious to me. *I should be doing something*, I thought. I turned to the two-way mirror and mouthed, "What do I do?" to my supervisor watching me.

She came in and advised, "Well, just play with him." I didn't know how to play with a two-year-old. I didn't remember being two and what I enjoyed at that age. Besides, this kid was doing quite well without me. The tiny one was bouncing around the room, touching this and touching that, and basically ignoring me. So I watched him. I tried to make contact again.

"My name is Miss Lydia—what's yours?"

Nothing. The little person went about his business, impervious to me, leaving me feeling very *inadequate*. I didn't know how to engage him. I knew nothing about this species of folk. I had no control, no power. My supervisor didn't understand my inability to come up with a thought about the nature of this child's communication. This child did not read the same textbooks I had just completed and been tested on. How could I evaluate his language deficits if there was no apparent communication between us? I started having second thoughts about the time I put into my master's level studies. Is this what speech therapy is all about? I began to think that I had obviously made the wrong career choice.

After I completed my bachelor's degree in theatre at New York University in 1969, I looked into further study at Yale University. I applied and was accepted into their prestigious master's level drama school. I wanted to be *the* lighting designer on Broadway. Ever impulsive with no clear view of the future, I blew the money I had saved for my master's work at Yale on an extended trip to Europe. I couldn't imagine spending another minute in a classroom. I was off for an adventure. On my return, I took a job at MCA Records (then Decca) just because The Who was signed with them. It seemed like fun. Clearly this seemed like a solid career move.

I signed on in the creative services department and designed album covers (remember albums?), wrote liner notes as well as internal publications, and supervised photographers at rock concerts. Basically, I got free admission and got to be backstage and mingle with the rock stars. I had a ball.

I met and partied with many well-known celebrities. Rick Nelson and Neil Diamond were a lot taller than I imagined. Paul Newman, whom I rode the elevator with each day, was disappointingly shorter. I shared my floor on Park Avenue with Paul Simon. Oleg Cassini got his breakfast muffins from the same deli as I did.

I loved that I knew Elton John at the beginning of his fame. I went to each of his after-concert receptions and became friendly with his mother, who frequently accompanied him on visits to the states. I still called him "Reg" back then, as many of those who were close to him did as well. Our birthdays were a week apart and I marveled aloud with him that two horoscopes could not be more divergent.

MCA sent me to London in the summer of 1970 to bring back the fringed jacket that Roger Daltrey wore on the Woodstock stage. The jacket was part of rock memorabilia that was going to be auctioned off at some event. Before turning it over to my boss, I wore it pub-crawling through London. I met and went drinking with Janis Joplin at Max's Kansas City back in New York. I served a tea to two upstart British nobodies, Tim Rice and Andrew Lloyd Webber, who were, at the time, exploring marketing themes for their rock opera, *Jesus Christ Superstar.*

After two years, MCA Records relocated to California and forgot to take me with them. I used my friendship with Andrew Lloyd Webber and the wonderful Tim Rice to land a job as the assistant to the lighting designer of the Broadway production of *Jesus Christ Superstar.* It was an amazing, circuitous opportunity to finally get back into theatre. But I disliked my supervisor intensely. I was also not prepared to exhaustively work around the clock, and then go for several months before seeing a paycheck again. In spite of working for someone I despised, I loved being involved with the production. We rehearsed in a loft on Second Avenue before moving to the Mark Hellinger Theatre in October of 1971. Yvonne Elliman who played Mary was already signed with MCA, and I had met and befriended her before the show. I didn't know Ben Vereen prior to his channeling of Judas. We remained good friends long after JCSS closed.

I remember the Tavern on the Green reception to celebrate the opening of the show. Ben arrived fashionably late. He was dressed in a tweed Sherlock Holmes-looking outfit, complete with cape. And Ben made an *entrance*. He strode in, owning the room, walked right up to *me*, bent me over, and gave me a big kiss. That party was a-ma-zing! I spent the rest of the night boogying on the dance floor with Andy Warhol and Tennessee Williams.

When my work with JCSS was over, dress rehearsal was a memory, and the production was ongoing. I had to think about what I was going do now. Designing and hanging lights was grueling, backbreaking work. On the Broadway stage, unlike at rock concerts, the lighting was seldom noticed. Unlike actors, the lighting designer was just a name in a playbill. Besides, if I was going to make comfortable money, I would have to sign on permanently with the vile man I loathed or compete with him, which, considering his solid reputation as a recognized Broadway lighting designer seemed impossible. I reconsidered whether I had the temperament, the crassness, the moxie, the strength to carry off a job in the big leagues of Broadway. I decided to back off and look for something else.

I floundered around using the valuable contacts I had made at MCA, worked at this job, worked at that, did some writing and explored different facets of my very limited vision. Then I remembered that medical show…about working with people with strokes.

I was sitting in this little room in the City College of New York speech and language clinic with the toddler wondering how I made such a mistake choosing this profession, wondering if it was going to be different treating adults. The stutterer assigned to me knew more about the profession, the disability, the treatment than I did—he was a certified repeater (no pun intended) and still stuttered after seven therapists. What was I supposed to do for him? The schizophrenic? I was way out of my league.

My first externship, or term of unpaid, outside employment after completing coursework, reinforced my regret of wasting months in graduate school, studying for a job that I was clearly unqualified to do, and in which I was basically uninterested. CCNY first placed me in an externship in a "600" school for several months. That's New Yorkese for a public school for the emotionally disturbed and behaviorally unmanageable. (The "600" referred to the extra money teachers in these schools got for their efforts—a form of combat pay.)

I was assigned to a middle school. Great...emotionally disturbed pre-teens seemed to be a redundancy, not a population I looked forward to working with. It was quite an experience. My supervisor taught me to lock the door to the speech room at all times. The hall with all the doors closed and locked felt uninhabited. No pictures or trophies graced the walls, probably for their own protection. My mentor introduced me to an actual paddle that she kept behind the desk as her only recourse should her delightful charges get rambunctious. Our "children" were ten- to twelve-years-old and bigger than we were. They were unmotivated, uncooperative and noncompliant with our efforts to mend their ability to communicate. I called the experience "Combat Speech Therapy 101." I was glad when that was over. I left the 600 school feeling ever more useless, disgruntled and dissatisfied. Funny. Now when I look back on the day-to-day, I simply don't remember the kind of therapy we actually did there.

But I do remember one small thing.

A willowy, tall, preteen named Raffi, who had a severe overbite and accompanying articulatory distortion, was up for parent conference. We wanted to convince the family to invest in orthodontia. Perusing the kid's records, I found the mother's name, Cynthia. Under "father" it said "Rosalita." On another page, the father's name was listed as "Frank." None of the surnames matched the child's. The permanent record listed the child's disability as "ED" or emotionally disturbed. Aside from this little information, Raffi seemed like a regular kid—and an intriguing looking kid. Graceful in movement, he was the color of caramel with large, doe eyes that had a slight Asian cast. I had attributed his reticence to self-consciousness due to his lisp.

Before the day of the conference, I asked my student, Raffi who shared his home. The eclectic population in that school taught me not to assume an Ozzie-and-Harriet, two-and-a-half kid, typical household. He said he lived with his mom and his dad. I asked what each did for a living. His mother worked for a publisher, doing work at home, and his father was disabled and homebound. Raffi didn't know the particulars.

My mentor and supervisor and I met in the school's conference room with a representative of the special education department in that borough as well as the school's principal. Raffi's mother arrived on time. I figured her for mid- to late-fifties, which was odd since her offspring, my student, was a good forty to forty-five years younger. She was dressed casually, in fact, sloppily in baggy khaki-colored jeans, worn Birkenstocks, and layers of garments above the waist. Her hair was gray and haphazardly cut as if she had hacked it herself. She was large in body and personality, owning a booming voice and sharp eyes. Surprisingly, she was friendly, warm even. We kept the conference formal. We suggested that Raffi's speech, academics, and social life would greatly benefit from having necessary work done on his teeth. Cynthia agreed. The conference was uncomplicated, short and sweet.

However...I couldn't help but pry.

"Does Raffi have any brothers or sisters?"

Cynthia answered me with no trace of hesitancy. "No, he's adopted. When he was five, we flew over and brought him back from Vietnam. He was an 'at risk' child, born with both sets of sex organs. He's androgynous. Raffi was a little girl when we got him. We had to make a decision and because of our own situation, we thought it better if he were raised as a boy."

"What do you mean, 'your own situation'?"

"Raffi's dad had a sex change operation. He used to be called Rosalita and then changed his name to Frank. We knew the risks of the surgery, and that the new organ may not, well, function normally. Raffi's male organs are, well, they are tiny. And he has all the organs of a female including a womb. But Raffi's tall. He can pass as a guy and Frank has been a big psychological support to Raffi—man-to-man, you know?"

No, not really. I did not.

A month in a locked door NYC "600" middle school was more than enough to convince me I did not wish to work with a) preadolescents b) the emotionally disturbed or c) conduct disordered. Theirs was a world I had gratefully grown out of. The least of this population's issues was a lisp or auditory delay.

My next "taste" of real-world SLP was at the crown jewel of internship offerings: the Manhattan VA Hospital. Working at the New York VA was then considered a very nice job. And thus a career spanning forty years was officially born.

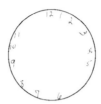

The Manhattan Veterans Administration Hospital

My next and last externship assignment was at the New York VA Hospital: considered a plum assignment and a prestigious place to work. The Speech, Language and Hearing Unit was on the eleventh floor, where I was exposed to a limitless number of limbless men, as our unit was next door to the diabetes ward. The VA campus nestled between the Con Edison electric plant to the south, and the New York University Medical Center, which then housed Bellevue Hospital, famous for being the first public hospital and infamous for once housing New York's nut cases. From our office windows we had a view of the East River and across to Brooklyn. I remember that my boss' basil plant loved the eastern exposure and grew to be enormous.

Medical speech-language pathology was then a relatively recent subset of speech therapy, having gotten geared up for the treatment of the military lucky enough to return from the battlefields but still with bullet wounds and brain injury. The Veterans Administration Hospital was funded to care for veterans of the Second World War and for those returning from Korea and Vietnam. Along with those who had head injuries, the VA was a long-term stay for amputees, psychiatric men, and a handful of women. Elderly and once-intact vets were now provided geriatric care including rehabilitation for laryngectomy and neuromuscular disorders, such as stroke.

It was 1974 and WWII vets still comprised the majority of the in-house and outpatient population. A small number of recent vets whose families lived on the East Coast were also treated at the New York VA. The West Coast of the country received the bulk of the injured 'Nam vets. The vets that lived in the NY area received their acute care in California, and then were transferred to our VA facility.

One handsome man got my attention even though he was pretty blotto by the time I met him. His understanding and his ability to express himself were nonfunctional. He responded with a constant forlorn, hangdog expression on his far too handsome, young face. He got clobbered by the rotors of his helicopter upon disembarking in the midst of battle, and sustained devastating and widespread brain damage. Puzzling—they must have scooped his innards and put them back in, because looking at him, the extent of the damage was not evident. He had only a fading scar across the top of his head under hair, which was already growing back. And empty eyes.

The bulk of the clients on my caseload were language impaired due to neurological diagnoses: head trauma and stroke victims. I had less exposure to folks with neuromuscular disorders such as ALS (known as "Lou Gehrig's Disease") or myasthenia gravis and such. I had a smattering of men whose throat cancer necessitated removal of their larynx. I had fantastic mentors and learned much about the disorder which lured me to the profession: aphasia.

Then as now, after graduation, the newly minted SLP with his or her shiny new briefcase, lab jacket and Lucite clipboard complete with monogram is expected to land a position. This starts a nine-month full-time (longer if part-time) Clinical Fellowship Year under the watchful eye of an experienced, nurturing, interested, mentoring supervisor. Yes, some of that is sarcasm—sometimes you win, sometimes you don't. No one ever explained why the clinical fellowship 'year' lasted nine months. If one would stop to think about it, this may be amusing to a professional group largely made up of fertile young women.

The nine-month CFY ends with a blessing from our national organization, The American Speech, Language and Hearing Association, fondly and familiarly tagged "ASHA." With annual dues and many hours of continued education throughout every year, ASHA confers upon the newly minted SLP Certification. This opens the door to a job, which pays just slightly more than what the SLP was making as a "CFY" and just about covers their student loan payments. Or not. Some of the medical SLPs merely remember and integrate their book work into treatment of the sick, others are truly born to the job. The latter realize they are dealing with fragile, devastated *real* people.

I was fortunate enough to remain at the VA after my externship there. After receiving my degree, I had been invited back for my Clinical

Fellowship Year. The New York VA Hospital was a turning point in the career I had been ready to abandon because I didn't have the desire to work with children. I vividly recall the men I met and befriended. Some have only faces—some have names as well.

Bert, a fifty-something WWII vet, was stuck in an aphasic groove, saying "Jesus Christ" over and over in a variety of singsong nuances and nothing else. He would respond to our questions with a variety of expressions of, "Jesus Christ."

When I asked, "Bert, do you need to go to the bathroom?"

"Uh, Jesus Christ Jesus," he'd answer, while his facial expression said, "no."

Bert, did you have visitors this weekend?

"Jesus!! Jesus Christ! Christ!" which I guessed to mean "yes."

"Bert, who was born on December twenty-fifth?"

He paused to think this out, then, "Jesus Christ!"

A broken clock is right twice a day.

I recall another gentleman at the hospital. He was being seen for a swallowing impairment. Until he was able to eat safely, he had a plastic tube fed through one nostril, down his throat, and behind his vocal cords into his esophagus, and then down into his stomach. The end hanging out of his nose was about eighteen inches long, and ended in a kind of rubberized funnel. He had sustained a closed head injury which rendered him "emotionally labile"—that is, he had no control over the manifestation of his affect. If he became excited or moved or saddened, loud cackling guffaws would escape unbidden and undesired from his mouth. He laughed at everything. When the laughter was at last controlled, he would apologize profusely. But he couldn't help it.

What he could help with was getting his fix of coffee. He admitted to a strong addiction to the stuff. So he would robe up, cover the tush that stuck out the back of his hospital gown, take the elevator to the cafeteria floor, and buy a Styrofoam container of coffee.

I had caught him down there once. "What do you think you are

16

going to do with the coffee?"

He assured me he was not about to drink it. Right in front of me, he uncapped the funnel thingy on his nasogastric tube, and poured the hot coffee into his tube. It was hot going into his nose and he yelped but then smiled with satisfaction. Between bursts of barely sustained giggles, he told me while he couldn't taste the joe going down, but he was able to taste his coffee burps. And he got his hit of caffeine. *Memorable.*

My supervisor was creatively trying to make our presence at the hospital felt, and we were asked to seek work opportunities in other than one-on-one contact with neurologically impaired patients. The solution was group sessions. My first group endeavor included methadone subjects—Vietnam vets who were once hooked on heroin and who were given methadone treatment. The program provided a chance to be included in an experimental communication group designed to work on grammar and syntax, but in truth offering them a chance to communicate. Really, the group was formed to provide emerging speech pathologists some sub-clinical, billable work experience.

I recall a bunch of young guys sitting in a circle, rolling their eyes at whatever speck of knowledge I offered them, courteous but definitely impatient to get out and line up for their cup of methadone. Each week the group got smaller and smaller, and soon it became a non-group. Clients with only a substance abuse issue and no other clinical impairment of mouth, lungs, or head don't make for a wonderful group experience. With the blessing of my supervisor, I made a commitment to form more gratifying groups.

With the fervency of the new kid on the block, I started many groups. I put together an aphasia group for men who were ambulatory or in wheelchairs. In terms of aphasia, they appeared to be a good match. I had visions of my clients helping each other, sharing experiences and being supportive. Joining hands, swaying, one-big-happy "Kumbaya" family. The group would have been successful if the ambulatory guys didn't physically threaten the wheelchair-bound men.

One man with a great deal of frustration built into his head injury—and a very short fuse—would suddenly lunge at another who was trying to verbalize his feelings, but had no adequate words and so would over-fix small errors in his utterances until we would feel like screaming, "Say it already! Spit it out!" I felt like a teacher on a playground except that the children were considerably bigger and less manageable.

I had a good group experience with my VA outpatients, one of which was "Jesus Christ" (Bert). These men had been coming to the stroke recovery groups that the VA offered for months, even years, and knew each other. My only challenge was finding topics then facilitating easier expression for some and interpreting what I thought was meant for others.

My least successful group included eight patients with left-hemi-neglect syndrome. Left hemi-neglect followed a lesion in the nondominant, typically parietal lobe and caused awareness of the left half of the body to...disappear. Other characteristics were a robotic flat affect, denial of any disability, and an inability to tell when one was touched. Kenneth Heilman, a neuropsychologist and renowned source for information on neglect disorders, defines the syndrome by what it is and is not:

> *"An individual with the neglect syndrome fails to report, respond or orient to novel or meaningful stimuli presented to the side opposite a brain lesion. The individual is not considered to have the neglect syndrome if this failure can be attributed to either sensory or motor deficits."*

~ *Heilman, Valenstein, Clinical Neuropsychology, 1985.*

I formed a circle with these folks who I thought would really relate to one another, given that they had much in common. At first many were downright friendly until I received the first complaint: "Why is he ignoring me?" Everyone was very social with his neighbor to his right, to his right, to his right, to his right...so that all my group members ignored his neighbor to his left.

"These people are very unfriendly," one man whined and stopped trying to chat. In retrospect it was very funny: one could approach the person to their right because they didn't know they had a left world, but that meant talking to *that* person's left side which was ignored. Oh well, I was still only a student.

The experience I received at the Veterans Administration served me for many years, allowing me to care for the very population I was attracted to while watching Harry Guardino in his role as an aphasic. The evaluation and treatment sometimes was the same each day, but getting to know my patients never got old. I dearly loved to hear about their pasts and admired their strengths. I cherished their successes and their return to fruitful living. I also mourned their demise. Fall in love with the elderly and they will break your heart by dying as a result of their ill health or long years—or both.

19

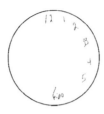

Max

Max was a crusty man in his 80s, who raged against his disability with an anger that may have saved him. Max was in the wrong place and time when two teens mugged him near his New York City apartment. He suffered a blood clot in his right brain hemisphere, which, in Max's case, affected his ability to discriminate figure to ground, to see in three dimensions, to hold his line while reading, and to comprehend letters. He became, essentially, dyslexic. Like a character in Sartre's *No Exit*, Max experienced his own personal hell: Max was an avid reader. When asked about his major goal with rehabilitation, he did not hesitate to say in his raspy Popeye-like voice, "I want to read again."

When he was evaluated, his reading skills were poor: Max was left with only a rudimentary ability to figure out which door led to the men's room and when to walk across a city street. Max navigated around his apartment fairly well. There was no bumping into walls or tripping. He lost his mild interest in watching TV. His hobby, his only pleasure was to read.

Max was a WWII vet who attended Stroke Club and received continued treatment at the VA outpatient clinic in Chelsea, across town from the hospital. I started treatment by working on Max's strong points. We covered all the basic speech abilities, understanding and the cognitive aspects of rehab, fairly quickly. His speech muscles were intact and working, so we began the journey to reading.

As I was a newly minted therapist, I could recall some of the techniques I was recently taught in my aphasia class in school. Now shiny, bound workbooks are available, designed, and published by fellow speech language pathologists—but in the 1970s we had only a handful of formal evaluations and the materials we assembled ourselves. *The Minnesota Test for Differential Diagnosis of Aphasia*, or the "Schuell" after the woman who published it, was my favorite assessment tool at the time and I asked Max to match an object to another one like it. We worked our way through black-and-white, bold-lined drawings of simple items, matching one to another. After a tedious eight weeks, we managed to match three-syllable letter groups made up of words and non-words (i.e. cat, hat, mat, dat, lat) to others.

Max exercised his visual fields by hunting for shapes and letters scattered across an 8½-by-10-sheet of paper and circling them. He looked for all the "o's" in a large print letter grid. Throughout the task, he impatiently grouched that this was "crap." All he wanted to work on was reading. He was a gruff man, quick to anger, and most of his anger was directed at himself. He saved a good dose for me as well when I arrived for his treatment. In spite of his behavior, I grew to respect Max—and his rage. "Baby stuff!" he would yell. "Crap!" "Shit!" One day, I just surrendered. Okay, I told him, pick out your favorite book and we will try to read it next session.

When I returned in two days, Max had picked out a white covered book titled, *Crazy White Man,* by Richard Morenus. *Good title,* I thought, *for Max.* It was about a man who quits his job as a writer-director for radio to live by himself in the wilds of Canada—a story of survival. The only problem was that Max could no sooner read the larger-than-average print in this choice of books than he could fly. Max was forcing me to get creative.

I made a template with a rectangular cutout that allowed only one line of print to be seen at a time. I suppose having only one line of print to see at a time was less visually noisy. I framed the extreme left margin in red to give Max's eyes a focal point with which to start. This helped some but he still had difficulties differentiating the letters from one another. I bought a line magnifier at a bookstore, which magnified and separated out the exposed line of print. Somehow larger letters were easier for Max to understand. Thus, Max and I struggled through the pages of *Crazy White Man* line by agonizing line. After sweating through several paragraphs, we would discuss the meaning, so we could enjoy what the book had to say. Max's comprehension of what he struggled to read was fairly intact, as was his short-term memory. I enhanced his day-to-day memory, reviewing the previous day's material so we could start anew on the rest of the book.

After 320 pages, which felt like an eternity, we celebrated

reaching the end of the book. Max had continually raised his own bar and now he could no longer say "I can't read." We closed *Crazy White Man* with much ceremony. I asked him what book he would choose next. All I got was a "hurrumph" and "Don't push it, kid." In spite of all the growling, Max was deeply moved by his success. His thank you was dinner out with my husband and me. This, too, was a coup for Max; leaving his apartment after his stroke for a purely social event, and this was first foray out into the world. I was touched, obviously Max's success meant a great deal to me as well. I cracked the code of dyslexia for one man, at least, and Max realized an impressive goal. He signed the book we crept through, line by line, and presented it to me for my own. It sits on my shelf today, a treasure amongst other volumes. Max taught me about pure perseverance toward a single goal. Max was a crazy white man, indeed.

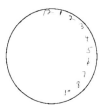

The Courtship

It doesn't matter if I knock at the door of a person's home or enter a hospital room, that first encounter is charged with nerves and curiosity, and when I know in advance the person is seriously ill, dread. My patients can be any age, from neonates to septuagenarians. My patients can represent any social or income group. My patient may be able to open the door and greet me—or not. Whoever my patient will be, the first visit has never hinted at the depth of investment we make in each other. I am always surprised at whom I become attached to—and awesomely surprised and touched by whose life I may impact.

SLPs are taught a recipe for that first visit: we announce our presence and the reason for the visit, introduce ourselves and initiate the formal evaluation. Depending on the setting, the evaluation may require completing a formal test or a series of several tests, presenting each item clinically and scoring the responses impersonally. Objectivity and observation are important: we never want to color the patient's performance. A seasoned therapist can size up a patient's needs more quickly than a neophyte and may stray from formal, rigid tests. If a person is nonverbal or somnolent, huge pieces of the formal test may be discarded and an impression arrived at quickly.

Graduate school never told me about the criers, the screamers, or the attackers. To sit down with folks, spread out the components of a formal evaluation before them, and woodenly recite the stimulus question while dodging punches or ignoring loud weeping seems insensitive and just wrong. Chatting is so much more helpful when evaluating a new patient.

Where are you from? Do you know why you're in the hospital? Do you know why I am here? are some standard questions. Sitting back while observing the individual while noting items in the environment adds so much more to the *totality* of the patient. And yes, we indeed treat the totality of the patient. Further, we treat whole families because when an individual has a stroke, a head injury from falling off a tricycle, some terrible disease such as ALS, or has been abused, each person involved with that individual has been impacted. The loved ones also have suffered the impairment—not just the individual. The mother of the kid in the pediatric ward, or the spouse of the eighty-year-old stroke victim married for fifty years, or the devastated grown children of an Alzheimer's patient who now must switch roles and parent their parent can attest to this. Brain damage is not a selfish thing, it gladly includes all who care.

The first visit should involve the family, if possible. Sitting, observing, and listening, the speech language pathologist can understand much about the patient before the brain damage occurred. Taking the time to establish a good history provides a wealth of information that may have slipped by the doctors or caseworkers. Discovering *the person* is certainly crucial in restoring that person to health or, at the very least, functionality.

Sometimes subtleties in the way a person responds to a greeting or conversation hints at the character of the suspected language disorder, or to an impairment in thinking. Language includes symbolic communication: speaking, listening, reading, writing, and gesture. It is generally recognized that language is basic to cognition in humans.

Most people think in a combination of visual representations (pictures) and in words. If there is a fault somewhere with symbolic language, it's likely that the individual's thought processes would be adversely affected. Given all that can impact mental status, the initial speech and language evaluation must include mental status testing starting with the basics: *Is he awake? Can he be roused?* This process continues to include the higher-level logic and problem solving tasks. Assessment needs to *assume* how the person's functioning was before the illness or injury. Some of the filler information has come from the history, some from the family, some just needs to be guessed.

The initial evaluation is the SLP's baseline and should be the patient's new beginning point. I tell my patients that their only responsibility is to be better than they were on the *first* day. Patients should only compete with themselves during each session. They should not do inventory on "goods" and "bads" *before*—or with their twenty-year-old self or with who they were in their glory days. The goal is to keep surpassing their own previous scores.

Traditional language testing starts with awake? alert? attentive? then checks all aspects of language: hearing, listening, reading, speaking, writing and gesturing. Traditional testing as taught in universities is rigid, timely, standardized and comprehensive—and seldom used in the real world. In today's insurance driven get-the-money medical world, every minute literally has value. The SLP needs to get in, make a judgment, write the plan of care then do whatever further in-depth testing as a part of ongoing treatment. Testing-as-treatment has value: one uses the same tasks as were originally tested so each day's scores can be compared to the time before.

The student SLP is introduced to several body systems: mouth, ears, nose, throat, lungs, and brain. The student SLP learns that she seldom works alone, that she is an important part of a medical or academic team or system whose purpose is to bring a person to wellness. The student SLP reads many texts, even more reference articles, a good many poster board in-services and listens to a passel of lecturers, confers with tons of colleagues, goes to annual conventions and gets bombarded with purveyors of the next great therapy gimmick or shiny new evaluation toy. And that's just for an undergraduate degree. Medical speech language pathology requires continuing on to earn a master's degree, which usually takes about two years beyond the bachelor's degree. The first of the two years is all about course work and tons of time spent in the college library or the Internet. Gradually, after course work the student SLP gets to observe actual therapy sessions. Finally, one gets one's own caseload and is closely supervised in the university speech clinic. This period of professor-supervised treatment culminates with an internship: a period of time exploring jobs in different settings— most of the time selected by the intern. Some of these people who attend the university speech clinics have had numerous SLP students and have maintained their patience if not amusement at us all.

25

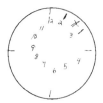

The Real World

After my externship at the New York Veterans Administration Hospital, I took a job in Westchester County, just north of the five boroughs. I bought my first car, a cute little blue Honda Civic, and drove opposite rush hour traffic back and forth from my Greenwich Village apartment. I lived in an apartment building on West 12th Street between Greenwich and West near the Hudson River. Three apartments were in the back and three in the front of the elevator entries. I occupied the middle-back apartment on the fifth floor with a drop-dead view across the rooftops of shorter brownstones of the newly built World Trade Center twin towers.

A Cornell professor rode into Westchester with me and I found him most mornings leaning against my car drinking his Chock Full o' Nuts (we were civilized before Starbucks). Looking up the block, I could see most of my neighbors sipping from their cups, waiting for their cars to warm up or for the first tow truck to glide by. The residents on our block became quite close, and we held block parties, or merely stopped by for much needed conversation in a city which could be lonely.

Westchester was, well, everything it was supposed to be— wealthy, stuffy, conservative, traditional. I lived in Greenwich Village, which had a reputation for being just the opposite. The rehabilitation hospital I worked at was aesthetically pleasing, situated on an old estate in a park-like setting, and I enjoyed the bragging rights of being a part of an internationally-known facility. Sprawling estate grounds were shared with an outpatient center connected to the inpatient hospital by a series of basement tunnels which we used on cold winter days. Underground was not as fancy as above ground; we had to duck to avoid slamming our heads on exposed pipes and ducts. An unoccupied mansion was also on the grounds, and it was used for after hour parties, and, I suppose, by the administration for conferences.

The rehabilitation hospital was well known and holding a job there was a privilege. I came highly recommended by my mentors at the VA Hospital as thoroughly experienced with all phases of neurologically involved adults with communication deficits. I quickly found that I knew very little about anything other than male aphasic servicemen and little enough about them. I had little exposure to any other types of impairments and there were many: hearing loss, spinal cord injuries, neurologically based imprecision of speech, Parkinsonism, cognitive deficits, and more. Because of the expectation that I was a very special addition to the staff, I adopted a self-protective, snooty attitude and basically avoided those patients I did not feel comfortable treating.

The rehabilitation center was housed in several buildings. On the other side of that basement tunnel from the hospital, was the out-patient speech department serving the adults and children of the surrounding area. Here was the director of speech pathology's office. An SLP specialized in the hearing impaired. Three other of my colleagues treated pediatric language and speech impairments. I had been hired to fill a spot on the newly-opened neurology floor in the in-patient hospital building. The other side of that floor housed the spinal cord beds. Before the neurology department was opened, one person handled the few inpatients at the rehabilitation hospital as well as all of their outpatient adults. Opening a specialized neurology section insured many more inpatients. I would be the second person, working solely with the inpatient neurologically impaired adults. And I was about to find out that a plum of a job had a worm in it.

The worm was my supervisor whose name was Miss Dudley. Miss Dudley was the person between me and the director of the speech department. She was friendly enough and I depended on her to show me the ropes. It didn't take long before I experienced the resentment towards me she apparently felt for not being chosen to work with the neuro team herself. I could not find any other motive for her actions. I had asked Dudley for guidance as to how to properly document notes in a hospital chart, as I didn't have to do this at the VA. I was also new to grand rounds and I needed to know what to cover in grand rounds, that important gathering of personnel involved with patient care to share vital information. I was clueless to my supervisor's meanness. She undermined me by giving me instructions contrary to what was truly expected of me.

I thought the workload a bit heavy and the procedures a little odd until the medical director—a neurologist friend of mine—wised me up. No, I was not to attend medical grand rounds with just handwritten notes jotted on scraps of paper as I was instructed by Miss Dudley. I needed to be prepared. I needed to type my evaluations, write progress notes daily and have information on all my patients ready for grand rounds where I would formally present each patient to the others on the neurological team. No, I was not to see my caseload and the adult out-patients—that was Miss Dudley's job. My erstwhile supervisor also insisted that I follow a strict evaluation regimen, using *her* choice of the several standardized tests available. She criticized how I handled one weepy gentleman. I actually felt her watching me through the two-way mirror. I couldn't get to the formal standardized test because my patient wouldn't pay attention to the test items. I chose to allow the weepy gentleman to weep before gently leading him to casually speak. I tried again to get to the dry, rote, academic procedure. The weepy gentleman sat and sobbed. I wanted to just sit and sob, too.

I spread out my test objects and robotically proceeded with item one: "Point to the toothbrush."

This produced louder sobs.

And in between tissues, item two: "Put your hand on your chest." Then, "Hold up two fingers." (I waited for the weeping to subside.) Onto item three: "What do you sleep on?" "What do you call this?" "Finish this sentence…"

Dudley told the director she didn't like the way I handled the session. I was not compliant with the Rules, i.e. *her* rules. What was I to do?

I remember thinking, *"Dudley, you made it to supervisor with your tactful, proper, political manner, with your managerial talents, with your knowledge of statistics and your expensive leather pumps and starched lab coat—but you don't care if my patient is traumatized. All you want are dry responses to stimuli."*

This supervisor kept leading me into minefields and I didn't know enough not to follow. This was my first job after my CFY, and it was clear to me just how green I was. I was constantly reminded of my shortcomings: it felt like home with Mom and Dad. Ultimately, I didn't make a wonderful first impression. Although I enjoyed working with my medical team on the neuro floor, including the head neurologist with whom I stayed in touch for years, working with the director and the rest of the speech department was becoming very awkward with Dudley as the go-between.

When my mother called and told me she needed me near to her in Florida, I decided to cut and run. Although I enjoyed working with my medical team on the neurology floor, working with my supervisor was becoming very awkward. After discussing things with Art, the man I had been seeing for several years, we had decided to move together to Florida. It was not a very tough decision to leave Dudley's park-like rehab center and not hard at all to leave Dudley. Years later I realized that every job has its Dudley. Every job has its minefields. Part of doing a good job is ferreting out where the minefields are, and staying out of the way of the Dudleys.

A B<small>RAVE</small> N<small>EW</small> W<small>ORLD</small>

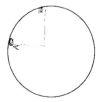

South Florida

I arrived in South Florida from Manhattan in July of 1976. My farewell to a city I had adored was marked by tall ships on the Hudson, and a fireworks display unmatched by anything seen so far. The year was marked not only as our nation's bicentennial, but by outrageous inflation—eighteen percent credit card interest rates and gas rationing. It was becoming more and more difficult to afford to live in the city. I decided to pack up my Greenwich Village apartment—the one with the fifth floor window overlooking the newly built World Trade Center Towers—and join my mother who had moved to Hollywood, Florida some six years before.

Only a fool would move to Florida in summer, during the hottest months of the year, but there I was with Art, my significant other and Phil, his brother caravanning down I-95 with all our worldly possessions. We left behind tall ships in the Hudson, Lady Liberty pointing upward toward unparalleled explosions of fireworks, and all of our friends. Finding a job was easy and, amazingly, the pay was more than I was making in New York. We moved into a small room in a two-story stucco apartment building that my mother managed, and I drove the twenty miles south to meet my new boss. The office was located on Lincoln Road on Miami Beach and it was headquarters to a handful of speech-language pathologists working contracts in the area hospitals as well as in nursing homes and home health. I was taken under the wing of a pretty, strawberry blonde, twenty-something named Sophie. We met at a local deli halfway between my apartment and the office and she filled me in on some of the details of the job that our supervisor left out. Sophie was the first (non-brain damaged) friend I made in my new life in Florida. I later introduced her to Art's brother, Phil, who had helped us move, and they later married and had two children. He recently died of lung cancer, a victim of smoking. Sophie and I still keep in touch.

The meeting with Sophie was important to me because, after only three years of work, during which I had the camaraderie of nearby colleagues to share questions and ideas, this job found me working alone. I went from hospital to hospital, house to house, and from one nursing home to another, alone. The challenge for me was managing not to devastate my already devastated clients. If I had a question, I could call the other women who worked for the placement company on Lincoln Road. Another therapist, Nora, met up with me and showed me around the two biggest hospitals on Miami Beach—Mt. Sinai and Miami Heart Institute. I knew we were fated to be friends—we both drove blue Honda civics.

We both also wore dresses and low heels. We toted our starched white lab coats in our cars to put on when we saw patients in hospitals. We were crisp and neat. I had no idea at that time how the job, how the clothes, how the attitude would change, nor how willing I was to get my hands dirty.

Since my mother had relocated to the Sunshine State years before, my boyfriend and I had a destination, a place to live, and I had a job. I drove down to the Lincoln Road office daily, was assigned a client, given the address (or name of hospital), phone number, and diagnosis. I called, made appointments, and navigated around South Florida with my trusty map.

My mother and I managed to get along. She prepared dinner for me and Art after which I would wearily crawl into our Murphy bed and fall asleep. During my days off, we would take walks, go to the beach, play cards, explore Hollywood, pick the fruit off of the trees that grew in our front yard, or go somewhere and listen to some good music. We also had a steady stream of visitors from up north.

Summer became fall and fall became winter and Phil came to stay with us for a week—which turned into six months. It was the winter of 1977, and he had stayed at home alone in Buffalo, New York, in his parents' house while they were in South Florida visiting us. In Buffalo, the snow drifted so high, he couldn't open a door to go outside. He spent time in the attic trying to keep the pipes from freezing with a hot water bottle filled with hot water from the gas stove. He ate cake mix—all that he had left in the kitchen. It snowed some in Miami as well that particular January—a rare occurrence. Art and I had moved out of my mother's apartment building and into a two bedroom on a pretty lake near Hollywood. Steve and Dorie—friends of ours from the city—flew down that winter and took us to Norman's Cay, a private island in the Bahamas, in their Beechcraft airplane. I was so impressed by Steve and this trip that I decided to take flying lessons. Learning to fly was a challenging, life-changing experience.

Lydia the Pilot

First was ground school, in a classroom with a textbook learning about TCAs (terminal control areas), dead reckoning (which is an unfortunate term for navigating by looking for landmarks), altimeters, elevations, and much more. After ground school, I hired an instructor and rented a plane. South Florida in the '70s had quite a few bases, small airports where private citizens could tie down their planes of various makes and sizes, and many flight schools. The booming industry back then (and I suppose even now) was drug running, and flight schools made a lot of money teaching up-and-comers how to get a plane off the ground, fly to a grass runway or levee in the Everglades, optimistically return to home base and then land the plane. Most people think flying a plane is very difficult. It isn't. Landing the plane is difficult.

Soon it was time for me to make my solo flight. It made such a powerful impression that I still recall the tail numbers on my little red and white Cessna 150. I did not take flying lightly. By far, it was the most difficult thing for me to learn—harder by far than getting a master's degree. I tried to practice flying at least three times a week. The flexibility of my job, on my own schedule made this possible. I would pick a destination, find it on a map, get all my tower and radio numbers written down and ready, drive out to the little airfield, rent a plane, do my go-around check list, and off I went.

Being a mile high or more in the air was indescribable. I loved flying by myself but if out-of-town friends visited, I'd bundle them into my little rental and show them the big hotels along the ocean, and Stiltsville in Biscayne Bay, where you had to search some to spot the wooden cottages built in a cluster on stilts above the shallow water and count the keys all the way down to Key West. Walk around for a while in this eccentric bit of paradise, then head back over the amazing endless Everglades where sometimes you can't tell the difference between land and sky. My days and evenings flying were wonderful. Me—alone—listening to the chatter on the radio frequency of one drug runner telling another where to drop "the luggage."

When I slept I usually had nightmares of what can go wrong (plenty) but these nightmares served a worthwhile purpose: they kept me careful during my flights. Fortunately I had few scary moments. But one time, I had just called in to the tower for a landing at my little airfield, and was on approach as instructed when a twin-engine red and black aircraft came out of nowhere and ducked under me at the very last second, so close I could see his wing rivets. I called in to the tower and reported my near collision and was told to file a written report after I landed. I brought my plane down uneventfully but when I tried to walk, my knees gave out and I realized how terrified I had been. The air traffic controller was amazed at how calm my voice sounded on the radio and gave me kudos for keeping my head.

Another time, my door sprung open at 6,000 feet and I had to lean out into open space to try to grab it. Luckily my seatbelt kept me in the plane. I could not bring myself to fly over water in a single-engine plane. Other pilots told me horror stories of losing the one engine and falling into the sea. These stories stuck and I never did take the plane to the Bahamas or beyond; however, flying over Florida's flat landscape to air shows, across the state to visit friends, or going to Key West or points north soon became old. Ever the risk junkie, I took up aerobatics. I had available, and took full advantage of, a 1930s, canvas-covered, red-white-and-blue biplane, my first love—a Great Lakes, two-place, open-cockpit biplane. I got to wear a leather Snoopy hat with a built-in radio headset and a parachute. I did rolls and loops and falling leaves and all matter of stunts, which I still dream about to this day. What a rush! I *loved* flying.

1978

1978 was my momentous year. I got married to Art on the beach on New Year's Day courtesy of a patient's daughter's gift of a wedding reception at the Fountainebleu Hotel. We were married by a notary who was also a divorce attorney, and there was lots of humor about this irony. Shortly after my wedding, two women whom I worked with at the office in Miami Beach, Nora Petty who drove the blue Honda Civic, and Bree Schrager met with an attorney and drew up the paperwork to incorporate a business. We three became Petty, Schrager, and Winslow, P.A. purveyors of fine speech pathology services in two counties.

Two months later, I bought my first house, a respectable three-bedroom, two-bathroom on a tree-lined street in the elegantly named Hollywood Hills (where the only hill was constructed by fire ants). After the house closing, my spouse and I were sitting in the empty living room on the carpet. We raised a glass of wine, marveling at being homeowners in the peaceful suburbs far from our old haunts in Greenwich Village. Without warning, there was a tremendous pounding on the door. BAM BAM BAM!

I opened the door to see a SWAT cop in black and full-body armor with an automatic pistol on my stoop. He pushed me back inside and told me to lock my door. A glance out the window revealed an entire SWAT team. A man in my carport and another man in the bushes, with guns trained on the house next door. We had just met the lovely middle-aged couple next door so we couldn't figure out what was going on. We later found out that the middle-aged, suburban wife went to see her mother somewhere and the middle-aged, suburban husband, who had found himself all alone with nothing to do, took himself to The Daiquiri, a neighborhood bar. He found some female company, got drunk, and then brought the woman home. The woman's husband took offense and called the police to report a kidnapping and hostage situation. Hence, the SWAT team. When the police eventually got access to the house, they found the mister and his female company sound asleep. So much for the peaceful suburbs.

This was a very different place than New York.

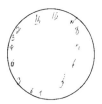

Nat

Shortly after arriving in sunny South Florida, I was given the name and address of a woman who lived a few miles north of my office in North Miami Beach. It was an L-shaped, elongated house on a cul-de-sac bounded on the rear by a river. The client's name was Doris and she looked like my mother. Doris had suffered a stroke and was living with her daughter, Natalie. Instead of quickly vacating the room when I started my evaluation of her mother, Natalie or "Nat" as she preferred to be called, asked if she could stay and watch. I loved it when a family member elected to be a part of therapy: the family who becomes invested in the patient's progress would be more likely will help with "homework" assignments.

When I completed the evaluation, I involved both Doris and Nat in my findings, my plan of care, and the likely prognosis for improvement. Doris' language disability consisted of a marked difficulty finding words. Regardless of her struggle to speak, she remained poised—at least in front of me. Much later, Nat confided in me that her mother wept after each therapy session for what she had lost and was not able to retrieve.

My first visit completed, Nat saw me out. Nat explained that she was a human relations counselor and specialized in death and dying. She and her partner were staging a training session for hospice and other end-of-life professionals that weekend, and invited me to attend. I did attend and that training session with Nat changed my life forever. Nearly four decades later, I recall Nat telling me to draw a horizontal line representing my life on a blank sheet of paper. Then she instructed me to bisect that line where I thought I was in my life. It forced me, at twenty-nine years old, to think about my life expectancy and, probably for the first time, to think about my future. Nat treated the subject of death and dying in an upbeat way, as a continuum of one's existence not "the bitter end."

Most significantly, meeting Doris and attending the death and dying course was the beginning of one of my life's most profound relationships. Nat became my best and closest friend. She cared for my well-being as no one else ever had. We immediately "clicked." We met often when I came to treat Doris, and then long after my time with Doris was over, and after Doris's death. Nat and I would meet for lunch and discuss peoples' peculiarities, her "normal" clients, and my "not-so-normal" patients. Nat, too, was a pilot. I thought it odd to befriend someone for other reasons and find we had flying in common. I enjoyed her husband, Mike, immensely and my husband and I visited their home for dinner and "salon" in the sense of artsy, European, literati get-togethers. Mike and Nat were timeless, so it was a shock to discover that I was only a year-and-a-half older than the oldest of their six children, and that there was a twenty-year age gap between Nat and me.

Kirk, the youngest of their three sons, was still living at home when I was treating Doris. Both Nat and I subtly avoided the discussion of age. I considered her my peer. Although we did not discuss our age difference, we did cover a wide variety of other topics—nothing was off the table. Nat and I shared the same moral code, religious views, and politics. I felt very comfortable asking her for her opinions on interpersonal relationships, and for possible solutions to big and small problems that I encountered. She listened thoroughly—a trait I considered very rare and very precious. She used her counseling background and threw the discussion back to me for me to find my own solution—rather than imposing her own opinion. She made me feel as if I were taking advantage of her therapy skills until I found her looking for my ear and my understanding. It worked both ways.

One day, she told me about a disagreement her husband was having with their son. Nat used this as an object lesson and told how she had come to handle her role in the situation. She admitted her desire to referee. But she backed off and said, "Mike and Kirk have their chemistry in a relationship that exists between just the two of them. If I impose myself into their disagreement, the chemistry changes. I have to allow Kirk access to Mike on their own terms. I have to let them come to their own solution." To that time, I had never considered the subtle and not-so-subtle difference in the bond that exists between two people that is different than the relationship that one of those individuals might have with someone else. And how the addition, or subtraction, of someone else alchemizes the dynamic.

Nat-plus-Lydia was not the same as Mike-plus-Lydia or even Nat-plus-Mike-plus Lydia. Nat demonstrated the respect she had for Mike and Kirk, and their ability to come to terms with one another without her. I encountered this idea many, many times in my relationships with my patients. I did not have the right to impose unwanted, unnecessary opinions or advice on an individual with whom I had a therapeutic relationship, or between that person and a spouse or other members of a family to attempt to *fix* it. I need only to guide my patients to alternatives to "fix it" for themselves.

Nat respected me and my relationship with her mother Doris and how I continued helping her with communication skills in my own way. After all, Nat must have had strong opinions on how to work with her mother. Nat became very involved in the details of stroke and subsequent rehabilitation because she had to be involved with the mother she took into her home. After Doris died, Nat stayed interested in the ways that stroke created "broken" communication, and its effects on relationships. As a human relations counselor, she had expertise in dealing with clients who were healthy and able to speak. Good, face-to-face communication was the very center of her profession. It was a natural bridge from using her expertise with healthy, speaking clients to dealing with communication in disrepair. So when I asked Nat if she would be interested in leading a group for the families of stroke victims, she jumped at the opportunity. One of my speech pathology colleagues led a group of aphasics (language-impaired stroke victims) in one large room of the hospital, and Nat met with the caregivers in an adjacent large room. Larger rooms were needed as the co-groups became very popular.

Nat and I continued to meet for lunch and an occasional dinner, and didn't always talk about our jobs. Nat and Mike were amazing amateur photographers who took their hobby to a high level. Their respective techniques improved as they softly competed with the other to get just the right shot. I visit with each of their photographs often as I am blessed with having each of them capture my child in magic moments. If my house were to catch fire, I would grab not only my son's photos, but also a blow-up photograph of a statue that Mike had taken at an art show that is eerily captivating.

I reveled in sharing the world through these two peoples' eyes through their photographs. I loved their freedom and impulsiveness. I giddily enjoyed a full moon lying with my husband next to Nat and Mike on the sandy dunes with the softly purring ocean close by. When ten years later, in 1988, I no longer wished to share anything with that husband, Nat reached out warm secure hands to lift me up and keep me sane through my separation, then divorce. When she realized she could not be impartial to the ugliness between my spouse and me, Nat used her contacts in the counseling community and gifted me with one of her colleagues who took her place as my confidant and therapist.

Nat lost her precious Mike to cancer in 1990 in their riverside home in North Miami Beach. Her friends and family gathered before, during, and after, and I finally met the rest of Nat's six grown children. So solid was the relationship between Nat and Lydia that realizing she had family closer to her than I was, I was not left out—the family just took me in. If Mom and Dad loved this woman, so will we, was their sentiment. Shortly after Mike's death, Nat decided she wished to be in closer proximity to the five children who lived in Atlanta, Georgia. Nat left her house to stay with one of her daughters while another of her friends and I packed up whatever the movers didn't take.

Nat and I met in 1976, and Nat moved, if memory serves, around 1991. Her relocation left us with a quandary: How would we meet for lunch? We solved the problem by having not-lunch dates and since we were not having lunch, we elected to not have lunch in very exotic faraway places, dining on expensive delicacies. We spoke often on the phone and during visits, but we made a special point of calling one another on specific meet-for-lunch days, like the day before New Year's Day. We would giggle and try to decide where not to have lunch.

Nat took her time grieving. It must not have been easy to lose a spouse as close as her own arm. Harder still to sort out the mixed emotions that come from that death: abandonment (anger), loss (loneliness and fear), and solitude (relief that caring for an end-stage cancer patient is done) and (fear) of the freedom of being in charge of just yourself. Her strong spirit allowed her to explore what more the world had to offer. She traveled the globe—watched whales frolicking, tortoises on tiny islands, and experienced exotic foods and people.

In her late seventies, bored with photography, and perhaps with championship ping-pong, she attended classes in stand-up comedy. Nat became quite a well-known stand-up comic, making hay of her "stage" of life and offering jokes with hilarious sexual innuendos. She tells the audience, "It's not easy being old. You have to depend on others to do things for you: a plumber to clean out my pipes, a guy to get the gray off the roof, and a gardener to trim my bush." She ends with, "If Mike could see me now, he would turn over in his urn and fall off the mantle." She memorialized our ritual by sharing with her audience how we met for not-lunch dates and the quirky places we thought to not-go.

Mike once told of a visit to a psychic who had also worked as a counselor. Nat also went to see him and agreed that Vincent was almost too close for comfort. Both said I should go. Vincent saw me in January of 1983. I recorded the session. The hairs on my neck still tingle when I remember all that he'd said. Among physical characteristics (the broken nose, the anemia in my youth, and my nearsightedness) and life milestones (my ectopic pregnancy the year before that had nearly killed me and my learning to fly), Vincent told me I would soon be alone with the child I was carrying. He said that Art and I were of divergent temperaments and not meant to stay together. He said I would marry soon after my divorce from Art. To my breathless questions: "Who?" "When?" "How?" Vincent foresaw that my next husband would be my soulmate. He knew only that his name had a letter 's' at the start but did not know if first name or last. Vincent was sure that this man and I crossed paths often, as we lived in the same neighborhood. So, in a six-degrees-of-separation kind of way, Nat and Mike 'gave me' my soulmate, Skip.

A couple years after we married, my second (and last) husband, Skip, my six-year-old son, and I visited Nat one weekend in Atlanta. She had made arrangements to go on a photography shoot in the Utah desert, but the woman she was going to go with had cancelled. She wanted me to go instead. I couldn't because I'd just started a new hospital contract. "What about going with Skip?" I'd said, offering up my shocked spouse knowing he would love to "develop" his own experience as an amateur photographer. Two weeks later, the odd couple, Skip and Nat, flew out to Utah and crawled around the desert with their guide, cameras around their respective necks. Both got a charge out of bold tourists asking if Skip (who was a quarter-century Nat's junior), in his boots and Stetson was 1) a real cowboy, and 2) Nat's lover.

I lost my dearest friend in 2009. She died heroically of a rare leukemia surrounded by her adoring children. As she became sicker and sicker, I discussed death and dying with her. She achieved a different perspective on the topic than she had when we had first met, those many years ago.

I still wonder if she bisected her life line in the right place.

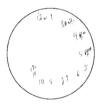

A Creative Solution for a Difficult Terrain

"A Creative Solution for a Difficult Terrain" was the title of a magazine article in one of Skip's model railroading periodicals. It fits the description of speech pathology.

I doubt whether I learned anything from my college courses that was useful in actually treating people. Rather, I see my contribution to patients or clients building on previous ones. Without shame I appropriate tips, hints, advice from one patient, solutions from another, and deliver this knowledge to the next client. I am just the carrier. With any craft, one needs to know the parameters, the fundamentals, before creativity can take place. Otherwise trying to create something without the proper tools is like digging a deep hole with only your fingernails. University studies gave me definitions of things, helped me learn necessary human anatomy, and told me where I could look for resources. It wasn't until I sat face to face with my first adult aphasic that insight occurred into what happens when people become broken. How are healthy therapists supposed to empathize with unimaginable disorders which rob us of memory? Of words? How can we put sounds in order to make words and sentences? How can we recall what each word means? How to get our point across or merely ask to pee?

Above all, university studies could not teach me the tenderness or finesse I would need to introduce fixing a disability my patient did not know he had. When something goes wrong with the very part of us that defines what is wrong and what works well, we are 'in the dark' to perceive what is broken. Add this to the denial that surely accompanies devastating trauma and a young therapist finds herself facing a client who has no idea that a therapist is needed.

The art of therapy is causing the least amount of psychic pain. The first meeting with a new patient comes with a jolt, an in-your-face introduction to the situation that he or she is experiencing. The patient is still unaware of the extent of his disability, in coma or in self-imposed denial, or in a state I call "nature's cocoon" before forays out of the ICU reveal the extent of whatever event has taken place. A patient is in devastation *before* the formal evaluation questions uncover a wealth of other stuff he or she can't handle. How the speech language pathologist handles this portion of treatment can either solidify a lasting, worthwhile relationship to build on, or, at worst, adversely impact the entirety of that patient's rehabilitation.

When I attended university—sometime after Medicare, but before today's technology—it was not yet fashionable to teach students how cognition occurs. We didn't really explore the strong relationship between language and cognition. Education in the public schools still emphasized rote memorization. Therapy was a prescribed thing: Do it this way. So sitting across from, eye-to-eye with someone whose brain is damaged, how are we supposed to know what is occurring *behind* their eyes? Our patient no longer shares with us an expected common reality. Their reality is somehow different. We read in textbooks and know intuitively that thinking is inextricably linked with language. How complete is this relationship between language and thinking? Can one exist effectively without the other? Some aphasics are very effective survivors. Without the intact speech or understanding they once possessed, they hold jobs, they learn to get around, they love their families, they care for themselves. Several of my clients have inspired the deepest respect in me. Take away a loved one and I can tell you how mournful and depressed I can be, how eloquently I grieve. I get solace from sharing and receiving sympathy and understanding. But take away the very words…

41

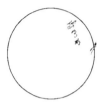

Bea

The address was one of Hollywood, Florida's finest: a large Boca-style two-story on a tree-lined street. Her daughter, Evelyn met me at the door of her home. She looked like one of those women on the afternoon soap operas that lounge at home all day wearing evening attire and heels. I, in my informal skirt and blouse, was underdressed. My client's name was Bea and she was an elegant lady who reached eighty-five years of good health before having a dramatic stroke. She might have died. Instead, she was left speechless with one workable arm, and unable to walk. She heard the people around her speaking something that probably sounded (to her) like Chinese. Bea, a widow, unable to care for herself, was moved out of her own elegant home into her daughter's. Bea took over the master bedroom, which Evelyn and her husband gave up instead of having her mom inhabit the guest room. I know I would not have made that sacrifice—my mother would settle for the guest room. Bea had her makeup put on her every morning, had her hair freshly styled, and wore her good silk *peignoirs* to bed. She was regal. Her family, on the other hand, was hand-wringingly frustrated with her. They could not understand her attempts to speak. Bea was, in professional shorthand, "a global." Global aphasia combines motor and sensory aphasia: the person has difficulty understanding and expressing oneself.

Bea's daughter would creep meekly into her own master suite and fluff her mother's pillows, or freshen her mother's water, or pat her mom's bedcover. Bea would suffer her daughter's ministrations for a while, and then crease her brow. Anger colored her cheeks and she pounded her fist into the bed. She would yell then start to cry, her behavior chasing her daughter out of the room. Bea's daughter begged me time and time again to please help her mother to speak, help her express whatever it is she had been trying to communicate to them. She hoped for her mother to talk again. I sensed they'd been close. I also

42

sensed that Evelyn was handmaiden to a very spoiled mother. I sensed guilt, resentment, frustration, anger—all swirling in the air in that house and it was difficult to pinpoint exactly who or what was the source.

I started gently by controlling what Bea would say. "Up and…" "Left and…" Or I counted with her or sang with her. Like a sculptor, I'd mold the first utterances into longer and more meaningful expressions. Bea would master one word then find another only to forget what she started to say in the first place. I took Bea to her limits, which, unfortunately, was not a long journey.

What bothered me most was the very obvious rage that I saw on Bea's face when her daughter or grandchildren entered the room to do for her. Was she upset because she was the powerful matriarch now reduced to having her ass wiped for her? Was she on the verge of needing to say something before dying? Were there lots of words? A lifetime of apologies perhaps? How could I tap into these words? How could I unlock her voice?

I was as frustrated as Bea's family. I couldn't seem to "crack" her. Several weeks into therapy, in a massive unprofessional fit of frustration, I emotionally expressed to Bea my own frustration and helplessness at not being able to help her. I told her how much it meant to me to come to her rescue. I ratcheted my emotions up a couple notches, *What* can I *do*?! *How* can I *help*!? Soon I escalated into pure theater, flouncing around the room, flailing my arms, acting out my inadequacies. From her bed, Bea quietly watched. At the climax of my performance she *thrust*, her left hand skyward with pinkie upraised. A look of utter triumph appeared on her face. This stopped me in my tracks. I stared at her. I imitated her pinkie-up gesture back to her with a questioning look and a shrug. She looked at her hand and laughed heartily. Holding out her hand to me, she appeared to be asking me to correct her. It hit me in a flash and I stepped back. I assumed a tall, haughty pose. I held my hand up as high as I could. To this elegant woman I presented my middle finger. I shot her a bird! I gave her a one-finger salute! I was rewarded by tinkles of merry laughter and an exhausted look of sheer gratitude. Then she imitated my gesture. And did it again. And again.

The door opened a notch. Evelyn, her concerned daughter, was peering in to see what all the yelling was all about. I invited her into the room. Bea sparkled from her bed. She smiled radiantly at her daughter and presented to her daughter her left middle finger—a loud and righteous, heartfelt, "F**K YOU!"

Bea and I were victorious. Her daughter was...appalled. Bea used her new gesture to shock everyone entering her room. She *loved* her new gesture. I frankly didn't care if her daughter was upset. I had given Bea a novel means of communication and by God she was delighted. That one obscene gesture unleashed some good—and appropriate—sentiments for some weeks afterward, so it was useful for more than just giving her daughter a piece of her mind. Bea learned no more gestures, she regained no verbal expression. I discharged her and moved on.

I used this technique sometime later in a hospital ICU with an unappealing patient, Paul, who, high on drugs and alcohol, wrapped himself around a pole in a one-car accident. He struggled and struggled like Bea to make his needs and wants known. He became quite a behavior problem for the staff. Nurses begged me, the speech-pathologist-cum-magician, to "do something—make him talk." Always a mediocre judge of character, I was right in Paul's case: I figured before his accident he probably owned a handful of limited vocabulary and peppered his words with profanity. So I taught him to say the F-word. He picked this up very quickly and soon was able to start with this and tack on enough words to get him something to drink (f**k-juice), a blanket (f**k-cold), a backrub (f**k-hurts).

Ten years later I saw one of those faces in a restaurant that you think you know—but aren't sure how, or from where. The face stared back, probably pondering the same about my somehow familiar face. She turned back in my direction, caught my eye and smiled. The lightning bolt of recognition had hit her. Across a roomful of diners in a posh part of town, the handsomely groomed dowager with the familiar face triumphantly thrust up her middle finger and began laughing. Both of us laughed until tears came to our eyes. Bea's daughter nodded at me, I returned the nod with a smile and went back to my lunch.

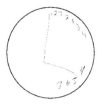

Bobbie

Bobbie was a thirty-eight-year-old, full-blooded Native American from Mississippi, whom I first met in her hospital room. In preparation, I knew only what I read in her chart—name, age, extent of insurance (just kidding), diagnosis (stroke), and referring doctor's name. Every meeting is emotionally and intellectually charged; my antennae were up to get every first impression, every sense of the person. Most of my knowledge of my patients happens in the first few moments.

Bobbie's first moments were unforgettable—she threw her teeth at me.

This gave new meaning to getting bitten by a fly. Toothless now, she was still radiant, but entirely pissed off, or maybe more beautiful because she was angry. Her high cheekbones were airbrushed red with anger. Her long, straight, black Cher-hair framed her large brown eyes, wide open and blazing, under Brooke Shield-eyebrows. She sat up straight in bed and I had the impression of just her in the room, but nothing else. She dominated, electrified the air. Bobbie was ranting. It sounded like angry ranting. She was hard to understand without teeth and she wasn't really giving out too much information.

Just throwing! Words! Throwing words! Hurling! Words!

What in hell had I done to her? I asked myself. *Did I deserve to have her inflict her dentures on me? No.*

Bobbie was *mad at* her dentures. Her husband later told me they both blamed her stroke on her dentures. They didn't fit well and made her nervous. Dentures.

Bobbie was a Wernicke, that is, a sensory aphasic. Like Anna, she had a loss of comprehension of spoken language because of a blood clot in an area of the brain. This type of stroke was mapped out by Dr.

Lydia Winslow

Carl Wernicke in 1908. I quickly determined that Bobbie was a Wernicke because her speech flowed and retained expression, yet the words didn't express deep meaning. She strung phrases together, repeated herself, and inserted clichés, kind of like coupling mismatched train cars. When I congratulated her on her flawless aim (the dentures nipped my ear), she tilted her head, RCA Victor dog-style and stared at me, her own words interrupted for a moment. *Had she understood anything I'd said?* I wondered. She didn't seem to. She covered this up with another rant. I got in her face, right up close so she would look at me, and then I introduced myself. She stared. I offered to wash and reinsert her dentures. She stared. I applied a sing-songy style to my words, and accompanied them with pantomime. *Wash your teeth?* I pointed to my teeth. *And put them in?* I pointed to her mouth. Ah, a smile and a nod.

After this bit of business with the dentures, her lunch tray arrived and was placed on the table in front of her. It was hot dog day and Bobbie, apparently very hungry—or a huge fan of undercooked beige hospital hot dogs—leaned forward to double-handedly pick hers up. One hand made it, her left one, but her dominant hand did not. Her right arm hung limply, heavily at her side. Her left hand didn't miss a beat, picked up the hot dog, and pointed it at her mouth. She took a bite, decided she wanted mustard, and figuring out that that damn right arm wasn't the least bit of good, tried to open the plastic packet using her teeth, which as we discovered didn't work worth a dang either. Here's when I find out what Bobbie was really made of.

As I reached out to take the packet of mustard, to open it for her, Bobbie grabbed it out of my hand, presented me with firm loud gibberish and somehow bit open the mustard packet and helter-skeltered her various plates and utensils. She didn't need my stinkin' help. I had an image of dog and cat fights in cartoons, bodies becoming flashes of color with an occasional recognizable shoe, arm, face. She was hell-bent on being independent, her own woman. Weeks later Bobbie would have permanent black-and-blues from flailing around, falling, being "capital-I Independent" getting to the bathroom. But right now, on our first meeting, I was amassing lots of worthwhile information about Bobbie. And I was in awe.

Toward the end of her lunch, Bobbie's head flew up, her food was forgotten, and she stared at the entrance as excitement lit up her features. *He* entered the room. I got to meet her husband. Kisses and hugs (he and Bobbie). Introductions (he and I). He wasn't impressed with me, not one whit. In fact, he didn't like me, maybe even hated me, and acted like it. When I bring him up to snuff on what has transpired so far, I do so in my sing-songy way so that Bobbie is not shut out, and he flips out, demanding, "You are not to speak to her like she's a child!"

I explained why I exaggerate my intonation and slow my words. He was not convinced a) that his wife had any problem understanding— or any problem at all with communication and b) that I knew what I was doing. I summoned forth supreme patience, firmness, and all the tact I could muster (not my strong suit) and explained in deliberate showoffy technical terms Bobbie's stroke and the damage to her language.

My well-planned session was forgotten; I was held in thrall by the force of Bobbie's personality and her husband's ego. I have a theory that one's recuperation from stroke rides on the crest of one's determination and that one's anger fuels that determination. Bobbie's anger and determination were enough to heal ten people's afflictions. Bobbie was going to heal, but right now, in order to help her, I had to handle her spouse. Her husband owned the room. When he entered, Hurricane Bobbie faded into a soft, warm breeze. It was apparent that she loved him utterly. It was also apparent that he lived for her. This was *their* stroke.

After a week in the hospital, I followed Bobbie home through my home-health contract. I was delighted to have some continuity with her. I liked her a lot. Her home was not the opulent mansion I envisioned, but a large, tasteful but modestly decorated place on the water. Bobbie refused any help around the house. She got around with a cane—her right leg was weak and clumsy, and her right arm could not hold weight. She made do. Any circumstance that occurred, she figured out. She was consistently covered with black-and-blue bruises from falling, bumping, ricocheting, bouncing. Tall, slender, and beautiful in spite of her physical weakness and lack of teeth, her Bobbiness shone wildly out of her eyes. I wanted to be near her. I needed to figure her out.

I played the role of therapist, but I also sought something from her, some lesson she could teach me. She and I laughed through our language sessions—we had loads of fun. Bobbie was anything but morose about her situation. She did a lot of shrugging: "Whatever."

I would let myself in their front door, yell that I was in the house, and put my materials on the formal dining room table. She would join me, always sitting to my left. Usually we were alone—her husband traveled much of the time for business. The time allotted by the home health agency was only forty-five minutes but I always went over, finding it difficult to pull away from conversation with Bobbie. When her husband was home, he was formal and distant with me. When her husband was home, Bobbie radiated even more brightly. She confessed once that for her husband, she painstakingly peeled the seeds from strawberries for him.

Bobbie was hooked onto the melody of language from the beginning, in her hospital room, and used the melody like a rope to climb her way to understanding the meaning of what was said to her. The piercing stares into my face, the knitted brows and the "say it again's" lessened over time until Bobbie could carry on a simple conversation. Her verbalizations became easier, a stronger conduit with which to carry emotion and intent.

Little things come to mind about those times when I reflect. Bobbie's older sister visited for a time, and her strong, Mississippi fluid singsong voice filled the house. She made me my very first tomato aspic, which I discovered I didn't like because of the texture. She mothered Bobbie to some extent, and I think she would have been the only individual alive that Bobbie would have tolerated being coddled by. Together, they made me family—someone who was loved and included in things.

I remember Bobbie showed me a well-sanded wooden board through which her husband had hammered a very large nail. She showed me how she could impale a potato or carrot on the nail to hold it firm and use her left hand to peel or cut. She taught me furniture walking: redecorating one's home to allow a person to get around without a cane by reaching for, or leaning against, a series of furniture pieces leading to a destination. She had fallen so often and laid there fuming that she figured out how to roll onto her good side and use elbow and knee to push to stand. Bobbie taught me how to fall, and then how to get back up.

Months later, Bobbie was due to be released from home health and language rehab. I made promises to stay in touch.

I saw her husband outside the ICU about three years later, and with the same formal distance, he told me that Bobbie had had another stroke.

She was here, and I didn't see her? I asked myself.

She was not referred as yet for treatment. I could not have missed her radiance had she been in the room. "Where?" I asked Bobbie's husband. He jerked his head toward the unit and wordlessly walked away from me. Numb, I reentered intensive care and searched first for my former patient, the beautiful raven-haired woman, the close friend, but then had to resort to reading the names on the doors to the rooms.

The bloated face framed in gray hair was unrecognizable. Bobbie did not rouse to her name. The laughing, warm, deep brown eyes remained closed. For the first time, the lack of teeth pulled in the always-smiling lips. My Bobbie friend looked eighty years old. There was nothing for me to do because she was not a candidate for speech therapy at that time. I left her side in a daze. Her obituary appeared in the papers soon thereafter.

Bobbie was forty-two.

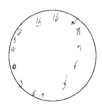

Contact Sport

Whether through boredom, desire for change, or because of the vagaries of the profession, which was financed in large part by Medicare (which had regulations that seemed to reconstruct every week or two), I have gathered an eclectic education.

Early on, I "specialized" in aphasia rehab. In the nine months I spent at the VA ninety percent of patients I treated were aphasics so I was not exposed to other adult onset neurological deficits such as slurred or monotone speech, or those hard of hearing who read lips, or those with dementia. After years of treating aphasia I...well...got very bored.

When I wanted a change of pace, it wasn't hard to find other positions in other facilities or contracts which placed me in situations where I would treat young, closed-head injured motorcyclists, divers into shallow waters, or fight casualties. Also, an ambitious, interested SLP could find many seminars offering thorough up-to-date information about various subjects in speech-language pathology. For the cost of registration, plane tickets, and a hotel shared by one or two colleagues, a therapist hungry for knowledge could shop and find most anything taught at a seminar—and get a weekend away from home as well.

These kinds of courses weren't an option—the American Speech Language and Hearing Association (which certifies SLPs and governs the field), as well as most states' licensure boards require a specific number of continuing education credits annually. One could specialize and treat only aphasics, or retool as a hearing impaired specialist or corrector of poor articulation, or work alongside surgeons to improve the lives of those with cleft palates or cancer. Today, interested SLPs enroll in Internet courses. We learn and receive continuing education in the comfort of our own dens. I was fascinated early on by a seminar on Sensory Integration given by an occupational therapist (OT) whose audience included nurses, Occupational Therapists and SLPs. I didn't understand much of what I heard then, but I had come to rely on that seminar again and again many years later at Sumter Center, and in the public schools.

Sensory Integration is an impressive concept of treatment. Sensory Integration (with a capital "I" if one refers to the actual treatment) means bringing an individual to a state of calm alertness by giving that organism's perception what it needs. Sensory Integration can be used to promote or extinguish behaviors so the person can learn by use of traditional teaching or alternative behavior modification. The sensory portion refers to involving all the senses—sight, sound, touch, proprioception (the sense of how one is oriented in space), smell, and taste. This is like the need to have a classroom environment at the right temperature, or blocking out noise in order to really attend to the teacher. Otherwise, attention becomes fragmented and people get distracted. S.I. has enormous ramifications to therapy, especially with people whose perceptions are askew (read here "autism.")

Contrary to the requirements of past professors and supervisors, and instead of immediately accosting my patient with a formal test, I sit quietly with them and trying to notice things.

Is the person peering at me, maybe feeling uncomfortable without the glasses she needs? Is this person cold? Are their dentures too loose and wobbling around and that's the reason I am not getting a verbal response to questions?

A patient once told me that she did not speak to me because she had to pee so bad she was consumed with the discomfort and could not focus hard enough to get the words out. She may have been labeled aphasic by an impatient SLP.

Before I can correct or teach a person something, I need to figure out if he or she is ready to work with me. Of course, it has become a comfort to have used the various formal evaluations and therapy materials. I can pick and choose consciously what is suitable for the moment without wasting the patient's time scrambling for material. I can jettison inappropriate, too-easy material for more material that is more stimulating, stuff that allows me to gain access to my patient's needs. As a new therapist it was very comfortable *not* to think of the person I was evaluating as a person. Just follow the recipe, complete the form, affix a label and put him or her in a pigeonhole.

I suppose because a good many of the people I sat across from weren't going to cooperate by giving me expected, textbook responses— they might sob, sit silently, insult me, even strike me—that I began to allow myself the luxury of *not* jumping right in. I found after many years and trials that I needed personal time with my patients. During this time, before the formal evaluation or therapy session would begin, I would try to crystallize an impression of a lifetime of habits, of the personality as he or she once was—and not the impaired person before me. Is it an advantage to have known a person as he was whole or to come upon him without the coloring of past behavior? I still don't know.

I now think it is useful to know about a patient's expectations and goals without foisting my own instead. As a young therapist I wrote the script for my patients; I didn't know any better. I had the control that they lost, after all. It was my prerogative to assume that I could tell this mature adult with a lifetime of knowledge and street smarts how he or she would comport from then on. What crap! The utter arrogance of anyone dictating another's path through life. For instance, as a young therapist I was appalled when a patient indicated or directly told me their wish was to end their life. That is, if I stopped to consider this an option at all. It took many years and many tears for me to know that my task was, most crucially, to guide, to comfort, to challenge, and to cheerlead.

It is a very personal thing, "an economy of effort." I always term it this way: What is the patient willing to put into what he or she gets out? My patients have taught me about the pleasure and appropriateness of merely sitting and gazing out a window, listening perhaps to one's evolving thoughts or reliving precious memories. When I'm old, please don't force me to play bingo or attend a current events group or do stupid rote therapy crap. Let me sleep late. If I'm rocking and looking out the window, don't inflict yourself upon me. If I spontaneously do a few dance steps or attempt some wit, don't quickly label me "nuts" and assume I'm ready for the dreaded locked unit. Get to know me. Realize that the person inside the old wrinkled exterior cruelly doesn't match the mind within. That despite an arm or leg that no longer works, or an eye that droops or a mouth that drools, there is still lust. Passion. Imagine! Talk to me as you would have when I was young and healthy. Inside I haven't changed. I might feel foolish because my hair isn't quite clean and my roots have grown out—or worse because I can't control my urine—but I am still the same person. Aren't I?

I'll tell you young people a secret: your patient's ancient, wrinkled, prune-of-a-face hides a twenty-year-old (or in my case, a thirty-two-year-old) soul. Call it a case of arrested internal development. And it seems to be universal. Every senior citizen I ask says they feel and think younger than their age. They flirt, they care about makeup, they laugh. The mirror lies.

Sensory Integration was one of the more interesting detours in my profession. Learning about deglutition—the not-so-simple act of eating—was another. I supposed that nurses have always asked for advice from speech pathologists about how to handle, or what to feed, a patient who has had issues with choking. Early on, swallowing had been a nursing concern; that is, nurses would need to figure out how to feed a person who couldn't eat. Then, occupational therapists became involved in mealtime because this group of therapists specializes in restoring a person's ability to care for oneself. The distinction is sometimes made that the physical therapists (PTs) and occupational therapists divide the body in half; the PTs work from the waist down on legs, while the OTs work from the waist up and with arms. OTs help a patient get food from the plate into their mouths.

With more and more research about the anatomy, physiology, and the breakdown of eating, the act of getting food in the mouth and down into the stomach became rather sophisticated. Technology was introduced to examine swallowing from the inside. OTs and SLPs then specialized by dividing the body; the SLPs worked from the neck up, and OTs remained an integral part of the mealtime team. They evaluated hand-to-mouth dynamics and supplied needed adaptive equipment such as padded or weighted utensils. Early on, I recall the turf wars between the OTs and SLPs about who was responsible, who had the most knowledge about mealtime. Who would get the segment of patients with swallowing disorders that had once been the responsibility of nurses? If I wanted to keep up with the demands of speech pathology, I had to learn about swallowing. Something I've done, well, all of my life and took very much for granted.

In the mid-1980s I worked in a hospital that used cinefluoroscopy to evaluate swallowing. The patient was brought down to the radiology suite and positioned sitting up between the two bulky parts of the fluoroscopy machine. She was fed soft solids and water mixed generously with a chalky-textured barium paste. The radiologist captured still, sequential X-rays of the patient swallowing, sort of like the cells of cartoons.

The SLP then looked through the static, fuzzy, black-and-white shadowed pictures, comparing one frame to the next, for any abnormalities in the rapid and continuous dynamic of the swallow. The radiologists who weren't in a hurry and were willing to teach a therapist explained what was supposed to be seen in each frame. Hungry for more knowledge, I signed up for one after another of the many seminars that were being given for the study of the breakdown of swallowing called Dysphagia.

I learned that cinefluoroscopy was giving way to videofluoroscopy, and that otolaryngologist (ENTs) were using endoscopy to study the nose and throat. Endoscopy is the use of a skinny flexible tube attached to a camera and a light source. To study swallowing, the endoscopy tube is inserted ever-so-carefully into the patient's nose, downward, and then stopped at the base of the tongue. To get hands-on up-close experience, I watched every ENT I could, and every SLP I encountered as they performed endoscopies and videofluoroscopic swallow studies. When I referred a patient with a suspected swallowing problem to a colleague who performed the swallow study, I invited myself in to watch. I asked questions. I got answers and was feeling pretty sure I could step up and do my own swallow studies. Many years earlier, I had attended seminars on video swallow studies and felt confident I could perform them, but I never had hands-on experience.

I researched the ethical guidelines for the performance of videofluoroscopic swallow studies put out by ASHA at that time. I discovered that experience under the tutelage of a mentor was encouraged by ASHA and by the professionals whose seminars educated us. No 'minimum number' of procedures or hours was stated. If I was going to get the necessary hands-on experience I'd have to step up and begin. Remembering how exhilarating, yet scary, it felt the first time I soloed in a tiny two-seater Cessna not that long before, I knew it would feel the same the first time I 'soloed' in the radiology suite.

So when I received my next referral by a doctor to do a videofluoroscopic swallow study, I inquired with as much confidence as I certainly didn't feel where in the hospital's radiology suite the videofluoroscopic studies were done, and just did it. The radiology tech, the radiologist, no one asked me where I got credentialed or where I got my experience. I did okay. After that first time, I had the chance to do many studies. With the same respect I had for trusting my life and those of whoever flew with me to a tiny flimsy-looking plane, I knew the person whose throat I was studying depended on me to do important stuff. This wasn't a game.

Interestingly, at the time I was *myself* learning how to do videos, the largest hospital district in South Florida hired me to train and certify other SLPs in videofluoroscopy—a skill I had just mastered myself five minutes before. "Skill" may not exactly describe what I was doing. In the beginning, I was tap dancing as fast as I could. The first VFSS studies were tricky. Black-and-white fast-moving film of swallowing was difficult to negotiate. Everyone's anatomy is different and the bodily landmarks, such as the hyoid bone, were not always easy to see. One has to watch the food or liquid, the 'bolus' in the oral cavity (or what non-professional people call "the mouth") as well as the moment the bolus passes over the tongue and into the throat. The bolus is visible in the video because it is mixed with barium, which gives it density and it shows up as black on the video screen. My earliest videos were a reminder of my cinefluoroscopy experience. Back then I had no ability to slow down the action so I had to keep my eyes peeled to see if that rascal bolus was going the right way or the wrong way. In some ways, the stop-action frames were easier.

Speech pathologists are joined in the fluoroscopy suite by an X-ray technician whose role it is to set up the machine, transfer and position the patient, wait until the test is complete, and then transport the patient back to the room. It is the radiologist who runs the fluoroscopy machine. The SLP explains the procedure to the patient, feeds the patient the liquids or solids, and then interprets the test and documents the results. Lydia, who was not so stupid, often turned to the radiologist and murmured, "Did you see that?" and waited for the doctor to tell me the information I needed to document a halfway-logical report. Occasionally I'd own up to the fact that I was inexperienced, and a favored radiologist might supply the information I needed.

The way you think your car can drive itself from its garage to your parking lot at work, do enough videos and it becomes almost second nature. I kept going to seminars and purchased DVDs of others' videos to hone my skills further. I did a ton of videos. I was favored by surgeons and other specialists who could choose which facility to send their patients for their swallow studies. I took the time to educate my patients and their caregivers, allowing them to see the videos and giving them a quick physiology course. They went home or back to their wards with solid information. If another SLP was treating the patient, that SLP would receive a copy of the full report as soon as I could get it to her. I kept in mind that my test results were a valuable tool for the SLP who was treating the patient. I never dictated treatment plans for the treating SLP, and I believe they appreciated this consideration. Doctors would be called and faxed a copy of the report about their patients.

One ENT referred an uncommonly high number of young healthy-looking people with no history of accident or onset of illness. They arrived as outpatients, sometimes right from their doctor's office. What I saw on the films was the effect of acid backup into the throat, or reflux. The effect was subtle and I had to 'stress' the person at times to diagnose this, tiring them out by asking them to chug down liquid or take repeated large spoons of solid food. Sometimes the source of the swallowing difficulty was obvious: when a person reports a lump in the throat feeling that doesn't go away, or a bad taste in the mouth, or wet burps. It could also occur when solid food had sat in the cranny just under the tongue. Or sometimes the swallow was a bit out of sync, due perhaps to throat tissue swollen by acidic vapors rising up—which could be as powerful as battery acid on tender flesh.

After receiving many patients who exhibited only the effects of reflux and not anything more serious such as a tumor or paralysis, it was time to educate the ENT who was ordering the test. In the hospital system, I held in-service training sessions for physicians who cared to come for the free lunch I provided and for the information on the SLP's role in diagnosing and treating swallow disorders.

One strange incident occurred between a referring surgeon and me. The patient arrived walking, looking as healthy as the people whose swallowing issues were due to reflux that the one ENT referred to me in massive numbers. This patient, let's call her Mrs. R—but I don't recall her name at all—told me that every time she swallowed anything, sometimes including her own spit, she would cough violently. Eventually Mrs. R stopped eating. She reported that she'd had surgery a week ago on her neck to fuse her cervical spine. I helped position her in the fluoroscopy machine where she nervously sat and stared at me while we waited for the radiologist on call to arrive to work the fluoroscope. The first black and white glimpse the radiologist and I had at the profile of Mrs. R's neck left us open-mouthed. Clearer and brighter than anything else on the screen was this shape sticking through the neck from spine *into* the woman's throat.

Neither I nor the radiologist had seen anything like this. We deduced it must have been the appliance that the surgeon used to fuse the patient's delicate neck vertebrae. Not just tiny screws and a thin plate, this sucker looked like dragon's teeth. I didn't have to go any further—I knew what the problem was but to be certain, I gave the Mrs. R a presentation of watery barium in a cup. I watched as the dark recognizable bolus made it back then like a waterfall flowed over the back of the tongue. As the bolus triggered a swallow reflex, in a milli-moment, her epiglottis rose and slammed into the metal appliance. She turned red then purple as she fought for breath and the watery barium continued its waterfall flow through the vocal cords and right into her lungs. After the woman regained her ability to breathe, I called her surgeon, right there, in front of his patient, from the radiology suite. I told him what we saw. There was silence for a long moment as I held onto the receiver and waited for Mrs. R's surgeon to, I don't know, tell her to come immediately to his office? Meet him in the ER?

After an eternity, he too-casually asked me, "So what should I do?"

Really? I thought. I said, "Sir, I'm a speech pathologist, you're the surgeon, figure it out."

One course I attended (which provided me with a weekend at Disney World) compared videofluoroscopic swallow studies with a procedure that was becoming popular among research SLPs called fiber-optic endoscopic evaluation of swallowing, or FEES. This course gave me the information I needed fifteen years before I, too, learned how to perform FEES. The way that I grew proficient in performing videofluoroscopic swallow studies, I used in adapting to performing FEES. I returned from the conference to my hospital with a solid education in performing FEES and searched for an ENT or other endoscopic physician (I supposed a doctor performing upper and lower GI's would do) to mentor me. I couldn't find one, so I dove in and stuck the endoscopic probe into the noses of any colleagues who would sit still. As with performing videofluoroscopic swallow studies, I gained experience by doing. I think I am now pretty good at both procedures and having both on my resume certainly made me a more attractive hire.

Of course, the treatment of swallowing is not all science. A nurse who was also a nun in a facility in Miami once told me that "quality of life" is more important than protocol. I've pondered this idea through the years. I have worked with compulsively by-the-book, very conservative SLPs, and I have worked with situationally-minded SLPs. If the facility in which the patient temporarily or permanently resides has protocols governing whether or not some aspiration or leakage of food or liquid into the lung is tolerated, the SLP has the latitude to allow foods in certain situations.

When an individual is hospitalized, the admissions clerk will ask if they have 'advance directives.' This informs the hospital what level of care they wish. They can choose "I want everything done" or "do not resuscitate" or most anything in between. One example of "in between" is "do not intubate" or "no feeding tube" and so on. Different health facilities—hospitals and nursing homes—have different 'code status' choices. So say someone has chosen to have everything done to save his life in case his heart stops or he stops breathing. If he can't swallow and if the medical professionals can't protect his airway, an alternative means of feeding needs to be discussed. A "full code" patient (wants everything done), has several options: very temporary would be IV or parenteral nutrition. Next option is enteral by nasogastric tube—a tube fed (no pun intended) into the nose, and down and around past the vocal cords into the stomach. A long term option might be a percutaneous endoscopic gastrostomy or a puncture through the skin of the abdomen. The doctor uses endoscopy to the level of the stomach to find the location through which a hole is made. A tube is pushed into the puncture and the endoscopist secures the end on the stomach side of the puncture—sort of like putting a bolt on a screw.

The patient can opt for a different code or full-out DNR, deciding that food is too important, even if it means there is risk of getting sicker from aspiration pneumonia, which can be a life-threatening condition. Doctors who have spent years treating patients with escalating debilitation become more permissive, somehow, with quality of life decisions. I have found this to be true, generally, in all the geographical places I have worked. The attending physician, and not the SLP, will be the one who will give his patient a can of Coke if the patient asks for it. And since the SLP works under the doctor's orders and therefore under his or her license, the ultimate decision on this remains with the physician. But, really, the decision is the patient's, then the physician's with the specialized input of the SLP.

I weigh the likelihood that I can keep my patient safe from the dangers of choking, against human nature. People are consumed with consuming. Some will be told they will drown if they drink and yet the desire to drink is so strong they will steal water or con someone into bringing them some juice or coffee. Make no mistake, since food equals love, family members will sneak love/food into the hospital room. Here again there is an art to working with human beings, the art of making possible a better quality of life.

You may think I have led you far afield and that I am no longer talking about brain damage. The majority of my patients who have experienced neurological insult have had to make these code decisions or have the decisions made for them. ALL of my patients have been alternatively provided nutrition.

To eat or not to eat. It's a difficult decision. I tell my patients it is a very personal decision and that it is my responsibility to provide as much education as I can.

An Alzheimer's patient who no longer can care for himself, who has forgotten his wife's name, and his children's as well as his own, who will sit and moan, but who perks up when it is mealtime: To eat or not eat? A terminally ill cancer patient who manages puddings and ice cream but loses most everything else down his airway: To eat or not eat? The thirty-year-old ventilator patient dying of AIDS with, perhaps, only a month to live, who never leaks food or drink out of her mouth or tracheostomy tube who enjoys a snack with her husband: To eat or not eat?

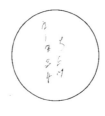

Shelly

Shelly was the twenty-one-year-old daughter of a nice, upper-middle-class family consisting of a mother, father, and two much-adored daughters. She was a year-and-a-half older than her sister. The sisters were very popular throughout their lives. They were both very pretty. They loved each other and were both very loved by their parents. The two girls grew into two lovely young women. They had their share of sibling rivalry, but all in all, they were close in age, close in temperament, and close to each other. There was the usual amount of clothes borrowing and copying of hairstyles. There might even have been some competition for boys, for their parents' attention, and for the attention of teachers and others.

The sisters were named Sally and Shelly. Shelly was the prettier one while Sally had the brains. Shelly began to date sooner, and soon began going steady with one nice young man. Sally may have been envious but she loved her older sister—they were very close. The girls' parents doted on each, but were also very aware that they couldn't play favorites. They parsed out all their love on both girls equally. It was best that way.

When Shelly accepted a date from her young beau to go to a rock concert at a nearby arena, things began to unravel for this nice middle class family. By chance, an approaching car had made its way across the wide median strip of grass and lost control. Its driver was speeding, and suddenly the late model sedan began to tumble over and over across the rutty median, eventually landing atop the roof of the car driven by Shelly's sweetheart. Shelly's sweetheart escaped a dark fate with only minor injuries—Shelly did not. She was rushed to the nearest hospital in a coma, the victim of a crushed skull.

She remained in the hospital for weeks in the ICU, and then on the medical floor, finally recovering enough and "medically stable" to be transferred home. Shelly arrived home many weeks after the accident, still connected to her feeding tube but no longer needing a ventilator to help her breathe. It was unlikely that she could appreciate all the fragrant bouquets of flowers, scores of cards sent, and piles of girly gifts, cassette tapes, and stuffed animals that were sent. All of Shelly's doctors warned the family not to get hopes up: Shelly's brain was dead except for the parts that kept her breathing and kept her heart beating.

Despite the doctors' grave prognosis, Shelly's parents and her sister continued to hope. They hired various therapists to work with Shelly. They celebrated every twitch, every reflexive eye opening. When I met Shelly, she was lying in her hospital bed in the center of the family's home, in what used to be their family room. Now it was Shelly's room. I had never seen her sister Sally there. The stereo played The Doobie Brothers over and over, the same track because Shelly's mom remembered that was Shelly's favorite song.

Shelly's limbs were contracted, that is, had become stiff with paralysis. She alternated between decorticate and decerebrate posturing. Decorticate posturing describes legs straight with flexion of the arms bent inward and clenched fists. The wrists and fingers are bent and held on the chest. Decerebrate posture describes legs straight with toes pointed and the head and neck arched back, with arms moved down and elbows facing each other. Both decorticate and decerebrate posturing are obvious indications of the severest brain injury. ("De" meaning "not" and "corticate" referring to the cortex or thinking part of the brain, and "cerebrate" referring to the cerebellum or the regulator of motor function, such as breathing.) Shelly's physical therapists routinely provided her with passive ranging of her arms and legs; that is, the therapist slowly and gently moved Shelly's limbs for her. This was important for muscle integrity and circulation in a recovering patient. But Shelly would not recover.

Unlike moving someone else's limbs for them, communication is a two-way street. One cannot "passively" communicate. The person in a coma is obviously not participating in any sort of interaction. The person in a coma needs to be coaxed out of coma. This was new ground for me. I honed my limited skills in coma recovery using Shelly as my guinea pig.

Coma is medically defined as a state of unconsciousness. It is a medical emergency. Coma is understood by some to mean a deep sleep, a sleep from which one can't be roused by shaking or setting an alarm. There are levels of coma measured routinely by a neurological instrument called the [1]Glascow Coma Scale.

Originally published to reliably and objectively quantify the status of a person's nervous system following head injury, the Glascow Coma Scale is now used routinely as a regular part of ICU protocol. The GCS measures three elements: 'eyes' with scores ranging from does not open to opens spontaneously; 'verbal' with scores ranging from no sounds, to oriented and conversing normally; and 'motor' with scores ranging from no movement to obeys commands. While coma does describe unconsciousness, it is layered in stages of alertness.

First I had to get any kind of reaction from any of Shelly's senses: sight, touch, hearing, smell, or taste. I lifted the lid of Shelly's eye to check her pupil dilation response and also to check if she volitionally tried to close her eye. She didn't. Sometimes when I examined her, her eyes were open. I flashed lights in Shelly's open eyes. I stood first at one side of her then at the other and observed if she was startled by loud horns or cymbals. Did she try to turn in my direction? She didn't. I massaged her hands and temples with aromatic lotions and oils. I scratched her head with a spaghetti lifter (this kitchen utensil makes an ideal back scratcher). I held noxious and attractive smells under her nose. I pried my way into the corner of her mouth and massaged her gums and tongue. I iced her cheeks or vibrated the nape of her neck. I did not know much about neuromuscular postures or about Bobath[2], an approach in neurological rehabilitation that uses re-education to regain normal movement.

Shelly was a cooperative patient: she rewarded me every so often with a reflexive grimace or eyes-wide-open. But it was probably not in response to something I did. At these times, her mother would run excitedly into the room and throw a little celebratory party for herself that Shelly was recovering. Yes! At last.

Shelly was my first coma patient and I gave her all I knew, including hope. She was also my first introduction to a family's agonizing inability to let go. Childless at the time, I couldn't wrap my head around this concept of holding on. Why keep this person, their

---

[1] www.brainline.org/content/2010/10/what-is-the-Glascow-coma-scale.html.

[2] www.wikipedia.org/wik/Bobath_concept

child, alive? Later in my career, I would meet families of all types, other families who would not consider giving up. Shelly's mother and father devoted themselves to her impossible recovery, and in the process cutoff caring for their other vibrant, healthy daughter. After an eternity of trying three times a week for months, I told Shelly's parents I did not see any progress and would not be back. They were paying me precious money and I could not morally take money that they might need later. The last I heard, they hired yet another speech pathologist to continue trying.

My time with Shelly stimulated end-of-life questions for myself. What do I want to have done with me, in the case that I enter coma and stay there? At what point does one call it quits? People come off ventilators and out of coma all the time. Some experience a fulfilled lifestyle with a cherished family, growing children, productivity. Other people, whom I would intimately come to know later in my career working in long-term acute care, never get well. Their fate has them going from one crisis to another, one organ failure, one infection to another. Loved ones are sometimes left hoping, stressing then despairing. End of life is expensive for the surviving family: financially as well as emotionally.

At one point does one let nature—or God—take its course and just let go?

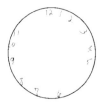

Sheila

This referral was unusual. Normally when there was a consultation called in to our office, a hospital would give us the patient's name, room number, doctor's name, and diagnosis. This time, I did not get much information. The contact stated that I was to see the social worker before approaching the nurses' station or the patient's room.

The hospital social worker had been expecting me. She sounded tenuous, hesitant and careful: very mysterious. I wondered what was in store for me. My new patient's name was Sheila S. I kept wondering why she warranted all this extra attention. Why was she so special? I was not told much by the social worker. Only that Sheila was a gunshot victim and she was the same age as Shelly, only twenty-two. So far this was not anything out of the ordinary for the profession, however, the social worker's mannerisms told me more than her words: "Read her history first." Obviously this case involved heavy dynamics. I rode the elevator up alone with both excitement and dread.

When I arrived at the room, my patient was seated upright in her bed. A wide ray of sunshine may have been streaming into the window to highlight her face. Or not. I may have made this part up. She was a goddess. She was so beautiful. *Be careful what you wish for* came unbidden into my mind. I wanted such beauty for myself and had no idea what strings were attached. And her head was bald and dented in on both sides as if by fingers poking into clay.

She followed my entrance into the room with her eyes. She was expressionless as I introduced myself. Sheila looked like a character from *Children of the Corn* or *Dawn of the Dead*. She offered nothing, no facial expression, she merely continued staring at me. I patted her hand and excused myself, assuring her blank, beautiful face that I would quickly return.

I could not imagine what would warrant the social worker's dire warning, so I read her medical chart. At the nurses' station, Sheila's medical chart offered some background. Sheila was a "9-1-1" in the late afternoon. She was found unconscious and breathing in a lake of her own blood, with a .22 caliber pistol lying next to her hand on the floor on the very same floor, in the very same room, where Sheila's mother lay some months before. Shot through the head, her mother was a very successful suicide. Sheila was not. It was Sheila who had discovered her mother's lifeless body.

Sheila had chosen a small caliber pistol, and the small, .22 bullet followed the brain pan (the inside of the skull which holds the brain) all the way around and then out. The dents in her head were a result of the surgeon's attempt to save her life by removing the bullet fragments and gunpowder residue. Sheila survived and received an unanticipated frontal lobotomy in the process. She looked it: emotionless, watchful but zombie-like, silent, and creepy. Stark contrast to the pictures of Sheila before her "incident" that someone had taped to the wall in her hospital room. In her photos, she has a big smile, straight white teeth. Her long, wavy blonde hair is parted in the middle, falling over her shoulders. Here is Sheila in a red bikini on the beach. Sheila with friends, laughing, arms around each other. She is a small, slender girl. She is a strikingly gorgeous girl. Before the "incident."

The head, deprived of its usual long blonde hair, somehow suited her. Her sea-blue eyes dominated and held you as she watched steadily, unblinking. An occasional sigh would accompany a switch of attention. Sheila's glance moved to the window, watching…what?

A nurse stopped in the room, as curious as to who I was, as she was about Sheila's welfare. "She doesn't talk," she offered, and then added, "but she understands everything."

How do you know? I wondered.

The evaluation took several sessions. Sheila demonstrated that she understood some things said to her. She lifted delicate fingers off the coverlet to show "one" and "two" to command. She very slowly nodded her head "yes" to the question, "Is your first name Sheila?" and as slowly, shook her head when asked if her name was Mary. She offered no speech. It was not a complicated evaluation. Sheila S. had a communication disorder—that was clear. And she needed fixing. That, too, was clear. I wrote up a formal program for her, wrote up her consultation report for her medical chart, buckled my emotional seatbelt and planned to see her daily.

I had so many questions. Was Sheila aware that she was alive? It seemed nuts, but was it possible that she did not know she survived? Did she remember her suicide attempt? Did she still feel so much pain that she regretted surviving? And most significantly, what level of pain must someone go through to want to end one's life?

I met Sheila fairly early in my career and did not know as much about cognition or psychology as I do now. Sheila pushed me to learn more about emotions—and the meaning of life.

When I visited Sheila for therapy, I felt I was talking to myself. She would watch me as lazily and steadily as a cat would. She gave me no clue whether she was feeling anything, what she was feeling, or what her opinions might be.

I found myself talking to just talk. "I used to live in Manhattan. What I really liked was walking home from the subway and picking up fresh food for that night's dinner. The fridge in my apartment was so small so it made sense to pick up fresh stuff from the sidewalk markets on the way. Don't cha think?" Sometimes I rhapsodized aloud over a graceful bird sitting on a branch just beyond the window. "Look at the beauty of this world. How could anyone think of leaving it? Isn't this wonder of nature enough to keep you here?"

My heavens. I was way out of touch with this level of pain, and especially with Sheila's kind of pain.

Day after day, I neglected my other responsibilities to spend more time in Sheila's room with her. When mealtime trays arrived, she fed herself robotically, without mess—and without apparent hunger. She changed position in bed seldom: wherever she was at the time seemed okay for her. An automaton—a young, strikingly beautiful automaton she was.

Several weeks had passed and I found I was obsessed with Sheila, until one day, she thanked me for my attention by verbally answering one of my random rhetorical questions. I was open-mouthed shocked. She looked so blasé. I reposed the question: again, she answered. One word, only one word. One word! It was the first word since she picked up that gun. I ran into the hall, tackled anyone I could to drag them into Sheila's room so I would have a witness to my wonder.

She didn't let me down. I am surprised today that I can't remember the word she said. It should come to mind like the milestone of one's child's first word. It was a milestone, for me, at least.

As days passed, Sheila spoke more often. She recalled nothing of her life before the hospital. She provided her name, and discussed her meals and the events of the day, always emotionlessly, always impersonally. "Doctor Harris...morning. Took blood. I cold before not now. Raining."

One day, a particularly handsome middle-aged stranger breezed into Sheila's hospital room much like a ship's social director who did not expect anyone to take him up on his activities but who was just doing his job. Sheila's look told me that she sensed someone new in her room, but she demonstrated no recognition, no emotion.

After kissing the top of her head, he turned to me: "Hi, I'm Sheila's dad." He placed his motorcycle helmet on an empty chair, but did not sit down himself. He dropped kernels of news about this person and that person on his daughter, and said everyone at her restaurant missed her. She stared forward, not reacting.

His sexuality filled the room. Uncomfortable with him, him with her, and the way he too-casually tended to her, I started to excuse myself to wait in the hall. But his obligation was apparently over. He said goodbye, gave her a peck on her head again, nodded to me, and then left.

Sometime later Sheila said in the middle of another conversation, apropos of nothing, "He screws anybody."

I was rocked. It was her first entire sentence, and the first indication of emotion—strong, raw emotion. But it was said with no apparent emotion showing. Sheila was in there. Someone was home but living in the house without turning lights on.

"Your father?"

But she was away again, staring at a wall. Was this gorgeous man a factor in Sheila's suicide attempt? With time, more information was added to Sheila's dossier, whether fact or rumor. She'd had everything going for her.

She had the face and the body any girl would envy. She was a hostess in one of Miami Beach's in-spots, one of "those places" with a line in front waiting for the velvet rope to allow them entrance. Her

67

steady boyfriend was devoted and eager to marry. Her father was, if not wealthy, then close to it—had a Porsche and raced motorcycles. He definitely was a factor in her fate. With my own dysfunctional parents and being solidly in the middle of the middle-class, I couldn't imagine what life with a father like hers must have been like for Sheila. And I suppose, for her mother, too.

Sometime in the third month since meeting her, Sheila had developed a cold. Her nose ran a bit and since she did not care to wipe it, I did this for her. The medical chart told a different story. She was displaying signs of neurological instability: her face would suddenly flush red, her seizure activity increased, she lost her desire to eat. Her team of physicians theorized she was losing cerebrospinal fluid out her nose, and not mucous from a cold. Sheila lived a day-and-a-half longer. What was left of the cerebrospinal fluid in her brain had leaked out her nose. Without the necessary fluid, the brain will not work.

Three months after her death, I was still depressed. I learned to be careful what I wished for.

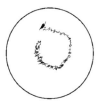

Leonard

The Bormans looked like those cute pilgrim salt-and-pepper shakers on the table at Thanksgiving. Both were equally chubby and sassy, seemingly satisfied with what life dealt them. You could tell them apart because Mrs. Borman's voice sounded like her glasses were squeezing her nose too tightly. Otherwise, they were identical. Since the mister opened the door to me, I asked myself why I was there. I checked my referral paperwork: Leonard (never Lennie or Len) had had a stroke. Really? I looked for evidence of a stroke that would render this man homebound for Medicare purposes (suffering an impairment which prevents the person from ambulating outside the home or otherwise being unable to drive or use public transportation for other than routine doctors' visits) and could see nothing in evidence. In the familiarity of his home, with considerable help from his wife, Leonard hid his deficits from all but the professional.

This is probably a good time to remind my reader that "speech-language pathologist" doesn't always mean just "speech" and that we don't deal with dead people. We used to be known as speech therapists, but then the formal title was changed to speech-language pathologists. The former title refers to the time when our profession was concerned with disorders specific to speech in the school system, such as correcting articulation deficits like lisps. In the medical community, the two titles are used interchangeably. In Leonard's case I would use talents other than treating his speech.

Under my professional ethics and Medicare guidelines, I could treat any communication deficit, which might include speaking, listening, gesturing, reading, or writing. In addition, because language is closely associated with cognition, speech-language pathologists may work as cognitive therapists. My education had encompassed becoming familiar with the brain and its geography; I had familiarity with exotic results of brain injury, one of the most fascinating of which was hemi-

69

neglect.

Leonard had a classic "non-dominant hemisphere syndrome." When a person suffers an interruption of the blood supply to the right parietal association areas of the brain, sometimes perception is adversely affected. In Leonard's case, he "neglected" his left side, just like my group of left hemi-neglect veterans who neglected the person to their left. Although his ability to express himself was spared, Leonard could not read and had discrete cognitive deficits. Because Leonard was able to walk, his physical therapist evaluated but did not return to treat him.

Leonard was rendered homebound by his significant perceptual deficit: he could not negotiate getting anywhere outside his home by himself. After initially meeting with the Bormans, I requested a specialist in the activities of daily living (ADLs), an occupational therapist, to see Leonard. Because the various personnel—therapists, caseworkers and nurses—are given appointments that do not conflict with one another, I was always left alone with the family. I did not have the benefit of having speech or neuropsychology colleagues around to discuss things that were strange to me, signs or symptoms that I had never experienced before. I had to figure this out for myself. I was determined to help Leonard as best I could.

He graciously welcomed me into his home, a large, sunny condominium overlooking the Atlantic, but although his words sounded genuine, his behavior was robotic and depressed. "Who is it, Leonard?" called his wife from somewhere in the back. "A nice lady," my patient replied. Although I called ahead to make an appointment and the Bormans expected me, Mr. Borman thought I was what? A visitor? A salesperson?

Later, upon formal testing, I discovered Leonard demonstrated what my textbooks had described as a classic neglect syndrome, otherwise referred to as left-hemi neglect. He saw nothing, heard nothing, and did not feel the merest touch from the midline of his body to his left side. I could draw a line from his forehead down to the floor and everything to the left of that line was, essentially, gone. A blockage of blood to a discrete area of a person's brain robs them of half their world, gone.

In our first conversation, Leonard looked way up at me from his four-foot-nine height, said I was most welcome to stay, and would I like coffee? I was a pleasant guest, not a therapist with a plan to treat him.

Neglect syndrome will frequently include a quirky characteristic: denial of any deficits. Leonard didn't need a therapist. He was just fine. He told me so.

"I'm just fine. Mom, get her a cup of coffee and that good cake you bought," he offered.

I felt strange inflicting myself on him. I searched my uptake sheet. "Right parietal CVA (cerebral vascular accident)." I conversed with the Bormans, over coffee (why not?), and performed an informal—yet thorough—evaluation of his functionality.

At first he seemed either rude or possibly deaf: he did not respond to the questions I posed while sitting to his left; his face remained still with no emotion evident. When I reseated myself to his right, he made eye contact and was appropriate, charming and well-mannered in his responses. He knew his name, he was up-to-date on some current events, and could verbally provide his address. Yet he had no memory of being hospitalized, returning home or having any problems getting around. I handed Leonard a sheet of paper with large-print short, simple instructions written on it. He glanced at it and declared he could not read it without his glasses on. His wife reminded him he had his glasses on. He shrugged, and had no interest in trying the reading again. I asked him for his signature, which he wrote with his good right hand. The left did not help to hold the paper down so I did. His name was slanted, blocky, and large with loops repeated and letters left out. He could not read his own name back to me. Clearly, as the informal evaluation was progressing, Mrs. Borman was becoming more and more agitated. She whispered to me that she didn't realize how impaired he was. She helped him wash and then dressed him because she believed that he would ordinarily need such help upon returning from the hospital. She helped because she loved him, not looking for anything that he may be unable to do himself. Revealing impairment in order to work with the patient to improve a skill was a difficult part of my job. I wiped my hands on a napkin, put my notebook and pen away and prepared to leave. Mr. Borman invited me to visit again; he had had a good time. "Sure," I said, "I'll be back in two days." I wrote down the appointment, made sure my session did not conflict with the nurse, and the occupational therapist and I left.

That evening, I received a call from the Borman's daughter, an only child, now an executive with a large hotel. She had questions. I described the session and filled her in on the dynamics of her father's case and his prognosis. She was considerably more intense than her parents, but she asked intelligent questions and appeared very concerned. This was a very close family. I asked for her phone number and told her I would stay in close contact.

During his six months of treatment, Mr. Borman never questioned why I asked him silly questions, or asked him to read, or asked him to show me around his condominium. With other clients, I explained every step of my sessions, reviewing the session before and sharing insight into progress or problems. Because Mr. Borman had denied his problems, I just started my work. My approach was nondirective with therapeutic communication and cognitive tasks built into everyday activities. First, I asked him for a tour of his apartment, which was classic. He walked to his right in a small circle, stopping frequently for no apparent reason and needing encouragement to continue. He frequently walked right into the wall or the left side of the doorway. He looked so cute when he walked. His little body was held straight with his two arms down at his sides. He looked above his glasses at me, towering above him. He reminded me of a little boy who needed a hug and I always looked forward to seeing him.

Initially, I had sat directly in front of Leonard, and then sat further and further into his impaired left visual field. I encouraged him to find my face and hold my gaze. My plan of care began by gently asking my patient to tell me his name, the date, his address, and other personal facts. Some days he had no difficulty, other days he was disoriented. As we reviewed his personal facts together, I wrote them down in big, bold, block upper and lower case letters. I used the techniques that I had learned with my veteran patient, Max. I supposed instinctively I felt that the "noisier" the left margin was, the easier it was to attend to.

I wiggled fingers in the left margin to call Leonard's eyes over. Then I drew a thick, red line down the page in the left hand margin. This worked out pretty well with Max years ago so I tried it again. I kept the lines of print separated from each other. Underscoring each line with a ruler, I coached Leonard through reading.

I told him, "Go all the way to the left until you see the red line. Do you see it? Now read."

Another exercise had him name ten things on the left side of the room. I monitored the progress of his visual field awareness by having him occasionally circle certain letters in a letter grid starting with large, sixteen-point print then progressing to smaller print. I assessed progress of his left awareness by noting how far from midline-to-left he was able to circle the letters. From circling the letters, we moved on to tracing his name, then copying, then writing his name without any cue from me. It was gratifying to see the evolution of Leonard's mental status and the awakening of his old abilities.

On one visit, weeks into his treatment, Leonard opened the door and stood in the threshold with one pant leg on, gripping his slacks with his right hand which his shirt dangled over, suspended from his right shoulder. He had his clothes on only one half of his body. My first thought was: *Where is your mother!?* After my initial amusement at my little wind-up toy with half his body clothed, I felt a stab of trepidation: *Where was Mrs. Borman? Why did Leonard have to dress himself?*

"Ma is still sleeping," was Leonard's explanation. Calmly he walked me back to their bedroom and pointed at his wife in bed. I sighed a huge sigh of relief as I determined she was alive and conscious. Mrs. Borman was, however, seriously ill and needed to be hospitalized. She wanted to stick it out as long as possible at home, not wanting Leonard to be left alone. I told myself this wasn't going to work. Leonard was in no shape to make decisions—neither how to handle his wife's hospitalization, nor for who was to help care for him at home. Their daughter was out of the country on business. I discussed options with Mrs.Borman. The home-health agency offered a temporary homemaker, a private duty companion, who would move in with Leonard until his wife returned. Mrs. Borman balked; a stranger wouldn't care for her Leonard properly—no one would understand. Not knowing how long she would need to be hospitalized, Mrs. Borman was afraid she couldn't afford to pay a private duty companion. Then I had a far-out idea.

My mother had met the Bormans in the community, and liked and respected them. Before I could stop them, the words flew out of my mouth: "Can my mother stay with Leonard? Would that be all right?" They were speechless, and very grateful. My own mother stayed in the Borman's apartment, sleeping on the couch, and tending to Leonard for the week Mrs. Borman was away. My mother had worked hard all her life, and now had no job to perform—she was happy to care for someone. She thought Leonard cute and charming; Leonard thought my mother walked on water. Leonard's wife came out of the hospital successfully, Leonard's daughter returned, and Leonard was none-the-worst for wear. My mother felt she did a fine job caring for "the cute little Jewish man."

Therapy continued, but somehow the atmosphere was different. The Bormans took little liberties with me when I visited, like having lunch or a snack prepared. A book Mrs. Borman thought that I might enjoy was slipped into my bag. I had just gotten engaged and they wanted to meet my fiancé. Little by little, over a bowl of homemade chicken soup, I told them of our wedding plans. Mrs. Borman delighted in advising on the details of my dress, my bridesmaids' outfits, whether or not I should have roses or gardenias. When I mentioned I had my heart set on a ceremony on the beach, Mrs. Borman knew just the place: secluded with a wooden walkway.

One evening, I received a phone call at home. It was Leonard's daughter. No arguments, no discussion: the Bormans wanted us to have our wedding reception at her hotel. All the food, liquor, hall, bridal suite, music would be on the house. Whoa! *Okay*, I thought. *No argument, no discussion*. Without her offer, we couldn't afford to stay overnight at her opulent hotel, never mind even consider a wedding reception.

I don't believe I will meet anyone who had the Borman's generosity or stature (no pun) ever again. Saying goodbye to the three of them when treatment was completed was very difficult. I was doing my job; something I enjoy and sometimes forget is significant to my patients and families. It doesn't impress me that they would be grateful. It's my job. Sure, I get attached and am surprised when my patients and their families do as well. Although I missed seeing the Bormans on a regular basis, I kept in close touch by dropping in and occasionally calling.

About fifteen months after my last formal visit with Leonard, I received a call from his wife: her Leonard had died, the service would be on Saturday, and would I please consider coming? I hesitated only because if I attended every funeral service, that's all I'd be doing. But I replied, "Of course, Mrs. Borman, of course."

I arrived late and surreptitiously slipped into the last pew at the funeral home. The rabbi was speaking of Leonard, listing his virtues and personal history. He went on to dignify Leonard's wife, his loving daughter, his sister and dear brother.

"There's a person I need to include although not blood family.

She is in some respects much closer, much dearer. I am speaking of course of Leonard's therapist without whom he would not have lived the rest of his life. She was invaluable in giving him back his dignity, in caring for him like another daughter."

The words were slow to register. I saw Mrs. Borman turn from her seat up front and gesture to me. Heads turned, all wanted to see who the rabbi was talking about. Me? Me? No one before or since has given me a gift of such worth. No one has ever thanked me in such a precious way. Leonard is with me still, to this day. He lives in my heart and his funny little image is included with his wife and daughter's among my own family in my wedding album.

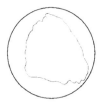

Daria

D aria P. was born and raised in a tiny rural village not far from Kiev, Ukraine. She had, I'm told, two sisters and two brothers, and they lived with their father in a large house made of a combination of what Americans would liken to adobe and peat blocks. The roof of their house, which I had seen in sepia photographs, appeared to be thatched straw. Daria's mother died when she was nine years old and she and her siblings grew very close.

Daria was born in either 1909 or 1912; both dates are listed on her formal papers. She immigrated to the United States in 1929, according to her passport, on a Cunard liner out of a northern port. She would have been between seventeen and twenty years of age, and experienced two decades of living with constant political upheaval in the countryside outside the Ukraine's largest city. She had witnessed, during her early life, the history involving two major battles in a revolution which greatly impacted the entire world: the Bolshevik Revolution which impacted the Ukraine in 1918; and the Soviet re-takeover of the Ukraine in 1920. Stalin's control had caused widespread famine and hardship, forcing many to leave. Later, when her daughter would question the two different birth years, she would explain that she needed to be over the age of majority in order to be sponsored for working papers in the United States.

Daria worked in the household of a wealthy gentleman and his family in Philadelphia, probably as a housecleaner or some such servant. He was her patron; he sponsored her visa into the United States. Some twenty-five years later she would introduce this gentleman to her daughter as her brother, Peter. "But why, Mama, doesn't Uncle Pete talk like you? He doesn't talk like he's from Kiev." She explained that Uncle Peter had left the Ukraine years before she herself had, and he had immigrated through Argentina before coming to America. The explanations came but were not always understood. Regardless, it would have been understandable for Daria to feel a closeness to Peter whatever their relationship.

Soon after arriving in America, Daria met and married a young man of twenty-one years. In pictures he was blond, slim, and very striking. She was likewise slim, brunette, and very striking. They made a beautiful couple. America was on the threshold of economic anxiety and, I suppose, that's why Daria and her groom moved in with his parents in New Brunswick, New Jersey. She set about learning how to sew and landed a job in a sweatshop making clothes. She apparently enjoyed her work and had several very close friends with whom she worked. That winter, John caught a cold, which had progressed into pneumonia and killed him. Daria was a widow at twenty-one years of age. She lived with or near her in-laws for the next thirteen years, sewing and involving herself with the fledgling Russian club in New Brunswick, which welcomed many of the immigrants coming over from a devastated Europe through the '30s and '40s.

It was in this Russian club that she met an older Russian man by the name of Jack. He had some degree of prestige, having organized and developed a network which worked to get refugees out of Bolshevik, Soviet Russia after the death of the Romanoff tsar and his family. Jack and several politicians and businessmen incorporated this network, R.O.O.V.A. (Russian Consolidated Mutual Aid Society), and parked it in its headquarters in New York City. In 1934, they also bought land in Cassville (a small town with a population of 307) in the pine barren coast of New Jersey, and established a community devoted to these refugees. They called the land Rova Farms: Rova being a derivative of the main organization's acronym minus one "o." I'm not clear how Jack, who commuted between New York City and Cassville, New Jersey, and Daria came to live in New Brunswick. I suspect it was because Daria felt a strong familial attachment to her previous in-laws. They lived for a time in a large, three-story next door to Daria's former in-laws.

A year to the month after they married, Jack and Daria birthed a little auburn-haired girl and named her Jacqueline. Rather, they planned on naming her Jacqueline, after Jack, but when the clerk in the hospital sat at Daria's bedside and asked her for her infant's name, she could not spell it. Giving up, she asked the clerk her name and settled on Jacqueline as the child's middle name when writing Russian, and the shorter, easier to spell Joan when writing English. But the clerk's name became the child's: Lydia. Daria was my mother.

When I was two years old, my parents, Jacob and Daria Winslow, moved to Cassville, New Jersey, to a tiny, four-room stucco house a mile away from the growing community of Rova Farms. My memories are of an icebox, a second bathroom—actually our outhouse—and an outside hand pump for water. I remember farmers bringing produce to sell from their farms right to our doorstep. The couple, who had made bread and pastries, came by once weekly in their aromatic truck, and I'd follow my mother out to make sure my poppy seed sticky bun was included in the sale. Milk was at the doorstep every week in glass bottles with bubble tops that held the cream as it rose out of the milk.

We had one of the first TVs, a small round-screened black and white unit, and, of course, everyone depended on the radio for news and entertainment. Pictures survive of this time, which show me at age three being given a bath in a galvanized tub outside, on the edge of our woods. Other pictures show me with an arm around my nephew, Paul, the son of my father's first daughter, and my half-sister, Irene.

The families around Cassville gathered with other Russian families whenever possible at Rova Farms. Rova had a sprawling white building with a wide boardwalk-style porch where the old people sat on benches and watched the people coming and going from the restaurant, the two bars, and the dancehall. The building was surrounded by green lawn and lots of lilac bushes, and the blue, white, and pink hydrangeas we called "snowballs." To the right of the main building was a lake with rowboats for rent, a dock to fish from and a grassy beach from which to swim. Near the lake was an outdoor area: an open-air bar and many picnic tables above which were strung colored bare-bulb lights. On weekends, we enjoyed bonfires by the lake. It was paradise.

On Memorial Day, like clockwork, cars and chartered buses disgorged Russians, Latvians, Estonians, Lithuanians and Ukrainians—all collectively referred to here as Russians—into the ample parking lot of Rova Farms. These Russians came predominantly from New York City's outer boroughs and stayed the entire summer in cabins and lodges that were part of Rova. The men would settle in their families and return for the week to the city to work. The women and children socialized, ate together in the restaurant or in communal kitchens, bathed together in communal bathhouses and enjoyed concerts, parades, the horsemanship of visiting Cossack riders, religious ceremonies, and dances. This was my summer life. My summer playmates and I were immersed in Russian culture, Russian language, Russian Orthodoxy and Russian drunkenness. On Labor Day, like clockwork, the part-time denizens of Rova would climb back into cars and charter buses to go home.

My father presided as the gregarious host of the successful Russian enclave. My mother chose to work in the restaurant as a waitress. After Labor Day, my best and oldest friend, Xenia, and I were let off the school bus and we would have dinner in the restaurant then do our homework together. Xenia's parents managed the resort and therefore, the restaurant.

It was the closest thing to a commune I'd ever read about, which was interesting since the '50s were all about The Red Scare, the Iron Curtain, Bolsheviks in every closet. The piney forests in coastal New Jersey around the epicenter of Rova Farms were inhabited by those who had fled and continued to flee communist Soviet Russia. Old retirees came down the hill from what we called "The Old Folks Home" to have their meals in the restaurant. Neighboring Russians came for the society: to have a quiet or not so quiet drink in the bar and then dinner of borscht, herring or caviar with egg and onions, and then chicken cutlet or stuffed cabbage. The children sought each other out and played out on the lawns or rowed boats in the lake. The adults surrounded the bars and got drunk. Inevitably voices would arise in a cappella folk songs celebrating the Russian heritage.

I have often thought of my parents as the original odd couple. They had very little in common—not temperament, not background, not vision. My father was sophisticated and sociable with a quick, ironic sense of humor; my mother straight-faced and serious who took pride in the experiences she accumulated, both as a youngster in the Ukraine and as a too-young widow on her own. She was street-smart, self-taught and tough. My father called her his "peasant." My father was a nonbeliever although he stopped short of calling himself an atheist; my mother was unquestioningly devout and a regular churchgoer. My father was very generous with money, if not with his attention. He worked hard and earned his money and before he could "squander it" (my mother's words) on drinks for his buddies at the Farm; she pinched every penny and threw them in the bank. I shared my father's looks, his ambition, his temperament. This must have irked my mother who just could not figure out who I was. She wanted me to be a miniature version of herself, I suppose. Things had to be done her way and she did not depend on discussion or anyone else's point of view. I recall loud violent fights as

79

the mismatched couple sparred to see whose view of the world won. My father soothed with alcohol; my mother used his empties to swing at him.

I don't recall my father doing things with me; my mother took me to see movies. The first movie I remember seeing when I was seven was *The Creature from the Black Lagoon* followed by *Jailhouse Rock* and *I'll Cry Tomorrow*—not exactly kid movies. I know who I get my good judgment from. (Sarcasm.)

I don't remember my mother ever wearing a pair of slacks. She wore the outfit of the times: an Ozzie-and-Harriet, Father-Knows-Best shirtdress and apron. Underneath she was literally straitlaced, going into town to get fitted for a lace-up corset someone told her would help support her back.

I thought it was a bit spooky that my mother generously volunteered to move into the Borman's apartment to stay with Leonard while Mrs. Borman went into the hospital for surgery. I found it out of character for her to think of someone else, yet alone a complete stranger, and not even of her own kind—Russian. But then again, there must have been much I didn't know about my mother, and much she did not know about me.

My father died when I was fifteen of laryngeal cancer, which had spread into his lungs. It was a bad time to lose a parent, especially one I needed to know better and had so many, many questions for him to answer. I needed him for my own identity, for my history, for the self-esteem a girl only gets from her father. I grieved with tears and powerful anger. With my father gone, I had to learn to live and get along with my mother.

I didn't much like her through my teens. I did love her and I did admire her, especially when, after my father's funeral, she climbed the stairs into the attic and brought down her old sewing kit. With my father's business closed and the savings used to search three states for a miracle cure that didn't involve cutting out my father's ability to communicate or breathe, my mother fell back on what she knew. She found a job in a sweatshop quickly and left me a latchkey teen.

I got on with my life, going to school, working, going to more school, working until the late '70s. My mother peppered each phone call to me with news of deteriorating health and psychological problems. I was ready for a change in scenery, so I left for South Florida to pick up my responsibility as an only child, watching more closely my mother's growing weirdness. Her judgment was ever more questionable. The people she was associating with and the way she chose to handle whatever money she had, left me uncomfortable. Long distance phone calls to banks and service companies and my mother's old friends who had also relocated to Florida, and whom she was slowly alienating, were sapping my income and my patience. In closer proximity, I assumed I could head off any disaster she created than I could tackle from afar in New York.

She had met and said she had actually married an Irishman so totally different than her, he was not remotely in her universe in background, nationality, nor temperament. He brought out her I-love-people-let's-party hidden side that I had never seen before. They seemed happy. The cracks began to appear when the Irishman reported to me that my mother awoke frequently in the night screaming about hiding in cornfields and Cossacks wielding sabers at her.

It could have been the time she admitted her third fender bender in as many months. When I asked her what happened, she shrugged. I asked for and received the police report for the second one and it reported she did not apply her brakes. She had broadsided a car when she ran a red light.

"Why, Ma?"

"I just wanted to," was her response.

Or it could have been her dreams, which became real, sending rats to prowl her bed and intruders to climb into windows and long-dead relations to mock. The once-fastidious, corseted, uptight lady, without anyone realizing when, had been transformed into a disheveled creature content to talk back to soap opera characters and dead relatives as she sat home day-after-day. I searched for a start and examined each behavior until even normal actions seem deranged. When did my mother become demented?

Dementia, Alzheimer's Disease, senility—these interchangeable words are enough to strike terror—and cause hopelessness and despair—in families. By the time such a diagnosis can be made, the patient probably wouldn't appreciate the significance of these words.

There were nightmares followed by episodes of falling. It would be only time before she broke a hip. As a medical professional, I could not ignore the fact that my mother needed medical attention. I knew and worked with many neurologists and chose one to examine my mother. After his examination, he pronounced her demented, "probably Alzheimer's." I immediately threw up a wall. No way. There was no way my mother had Alzheimer's. My patients certainly, but not my mother, never my family. The month before I got my mother's diagnosis, I was sure I had conceived and was in the very early stages of pregnancy. Good news, bad news.

I began attending all of the professional seminars I could, flitting from one city to another through my pregnancy looking for hope, for even a crumb of hope. I drew up a list of "hard" neurological tests and took my mother to several other neurologists and made sure each test was administered and considered. Alzheimer's Disease is tricky: the only sure diagnosis then was autopsy. Neurological testing merely eliminates other causes of dementia. The medical dictionary definition of dementia is wide open: general mental deterioration. The causes are many; strokes, hardening of the cerebral arteries, Parkinson's Disease, medication, metabolic encephalopathy, and other psychogenic factors.

Alzheimer's used to be called senile dementia or senility. Researchers have discovered that the effects and neuronal changes in the brain were identical in both and called both types of dementia Alzheimer's, regardless of the victim's age. My mother was diagnosed in 1983, and the education I amassed on dementia continues to the present. I now teach other professionals about the various types of dementias, including Alzheimer's and how to differentiate dementia from delirium and depression.

The hard neurological tests gave me no hope for my mother. I became an Alzheimer's victim along with her. In many ways, the families of victims suffer more because the disease blunts awareness of one's own mental deterioration. There is a bitter irony in that I could not see that my own parent demonstrated the same symptoms that I watched as detached as humanly possible in my own work. I looked over my chart of assessment items and knew I could never sit down and objectively evaluate my own mother.

Many elderly people fear that if they can't recall a friend's name on one or two occasions or misplace their car keys, they will fall into the black pit of dementia. In my mother's case, she never forgot names, she was not disoriented, she knew when the rent was due, and how much she had in her checkbook. But she forgot a pot was on the stove then forgot how to turn the stove on at all. Her dreams became nightmares and those nightmares became more and more real.

She forgot to eat and couldn't manage her medications. My mother had demonstrated a personality transformation. She became more paranoid. She was—all my life—somewhat suspicious, afraid that the Bolsheviks would find and torture her, but this was different. She was now whining, self-centered, wimpy, vague. Truth-challenged all of her life, she now brazenly lied about most everything, weaving enough reality into her confabulations to make her lies believable—and painful. When she spoke, she couldn't tie ideas together, or flitted from thought to irrelevant thought. She didn't know if she had spoken at all so that utterances came out of the blue or were repeated over and over again.

Her husband, the Irishman, covered for her, but I was grateful he was around so I didn't have to deal with her and her nuttiness. You can be sure I took away her driver's license—I just asked her for it and pocketed it. First, she just stared at me. Then she tried quiet rage, then not-so-quiet rage. I hung tight, and didn't return it. She got used to riding the buses or walking.

The Irishman succumbed first to a belly swollen with ascites, then from a liver dead of cirrhosis. Then, he was dead.

What would I do with my mother?

I closed up the apartment they shared and found her a one-bedroom close enough to my house to bike to. She was a block-and-a-half from the Sears mall, and I would see her doggedly walking to-and-from the mall to the apartment at different times of the day.

The middle of the night phone calls drove me crazy, leaving me an insomniac waiting for the next one.

"Someone's banging on my wall trying to get in and rape me!" and "A bird smashed into my window, I'm scared it's my father." And "I can't find my _____ (fill in the blank)."

The phone call I didn't get one morning was the one that changed everything.

She didn't call me and she didn't answer her phone. I forgot the bike and drove my car over in a panic. I unlocked her door and yelled but no answer. She lay on her bed swimming in urine and smeared with feces. I could barely wake her. I managed to get ahold of my husband and together we brought her to the ER. I called her cardiologist, a man who referred his patients to me over the years, and for whom I had high regard, to please meet me at the hospital and admit her, but he rudely instructed me to ask for a psychiatrist. He refused to come.

"She's demented. I can't help her anymore," was his only advice.

She was processed, cleaned up, and lay waiting in the ER for interminable tests. I was paged to the ultrasound suite.

"Do you know she has a mass?" they queried.

"Ah, no, what are you talking about?" I responded.

"We have to operate."

After years of working in hospitals with physicians who became friends and delving into one disorder after another, all that was erased by those four simple words.

"What the hell needs operating on?"

I was struck stupid. While I waited for her attending physician to conference with me, I stood next to her gurney and held her hand. She looked at me with eyes-not-crazy, familiar eyes of the mother that I knew forever, my well mother, my not-so-nuts mother. She said, "Please promise you won't let them cut me. I know what's wrong and I don't want them to operate. I don't want to live." I nodded, not knowing myself what was wrong. I mean, she was demented, and now there was a need for surgery, for a 'mass'?

It was Christmas Day, 1985, and company waited for me at home. It was the day after the ER nightmare. Her doctors intimidated me into signing consent for surgery, "You don't want to be responsible for her death, do you?" They had scheduled her surgery. I had close friends, kids and all, over at my house. Having the kids to distract me was a blessing until the day went on and on and on, and I was not getting a phone call from the hospital. Mom was scheduled four hours before, what's going on?

I excused myself, left the friends and the kids with my husband and went to the hospital. I checked in with the receptionist in the surgical waiting room and glanced at the other loved ones that had Christmas stolen from them. Hours went by. I spotted my mother's surgeon coming out of the surgery suite. I had treated this surgeon's own mother months before for a stroke she had suffered. He looked utterly exhausted. "She is just riddled with cancer. The mass began in her bowel but spread all over. I took out what I could and closed her up. And, oh, by the way, she now has a colostomy."

Colostomy and Alzheimer's add up to huge trouble. I took my mother to my home upon her discharge, ensconced her in my one-year-old son's room, and brought his crib into the living room temporarily until I cleared my head and figured out more permanent arrangements. The very first night I was awakened by who-knows-what. Every mother of a very young child has a spooky sixth sense and wakens quickly to see if anything is wrong with her child. I found my mother holding a package, struggling to negotiate getting out the back door. "Where are you going?" I asked her. "Out to dump the trash," was her casual reply. She was carrying my son.

Thereafter, I moved her back to her apartment and hired a companion to stay with her 24/7. She didn't keep her companions long. She drove them off by spitting insults or just spitting and being as difficult as she could be. Most of the time she just played with her colostomy bag, smearing poop on herself and anything else close by. My memory of that time was of overwhelming shit. I had a new puppy I was trying to housebreak, a young son I was trying to housebreak. I had a mother with a new colostomy bag beyond housebreaking. It was becoming too much. I invited her to take a drive with me, a short drive just to get out of the house for a little while. I headed for a reputable nursing home in my neighborhood and left her there.

Mother's Day, May 1986, stands out in my mind as one of the ugliest days of my life. I dressed my son up and took him to see Grandma. The nursing staff had dressed her nicely and put some rouge on her cheeks so she looked human. I saw her through the door of her bedroom before we entered; she had a spooky smile on her face and was quietly humming a phrase of music. *This won't be so bad*, I naively thought.

She heard us entering, ignored her grandson and snarled at me,

85

"Why did you leave me here Tatiana? You are a rotten no-good bitch."
She railed at her sister while looking at me, but didn't have a clue who I
was, nor who else was in the room. I felt the air go out of me. After long
moments of yet more verbal abuse I took my son and my clenched
stomach and aching heart and left. I wanted to save some part of that
Mother's Day for myself and my son.

Daria slipped into a coma the next day and lay curled in a fetal
position in her nursing home bed unmoving for days after that Mother's
Day. She had been a patient there exactly five months, having been
dropped off that January. I visited daily. I brought Russian music on my
cassette player for her to enjoy. I massaged her hands and her temples. I
brushed her hair. I held tight to her hand. It began to occur to me that I
was losing her and maybe what I was losing. My mother, for all that I
disliked about her, was still my mother. One to a customer. June arrived
and she lay still. I needed guidance as to how to proceed. The nurses
informed that they could not access a vein for an IV to sustain her. I gave
consent to forego the IV, knowing she would be dead soon without
liquid. In spite of our mutual animosities through the years, my mother
was my go-to resource for difficult decisions. I glanced at her in her
nursing home bed and decided, *Why not?*

I kept my voice quiet and asked her how she was. No response.
Then with my heart in my throat, I went on:

"I don't know what to do. What do I do?" I begged her. The near
corpse drew herself out of the fetal position, propped herself up on an
elbow and looked in my eyes. Her eyes seemed to gleam. They were not
the faded green-gray they used to be, but now the brightest sea green,
grass green, green of all the earth and universe. And they looked into my
own eyes.

"What do you need to know?" she asked in her own voice, the
voice I knew to be her own voice.

"Are you in pain?"

"No. No pain."

"But you have a huge hole in your back and I can see your spine.
It doesn't hurt?"

"No. I feel no pain."

"You are very sick. Are you dying, dying soon?

"I will die in three weeks, on June 21."

"What do you want me to do, er, I mean, what kind of burial, or funeral?

"I already made my arrangements. Dress me in the dress I wore for your wedding. Have the funeral dinner at Rova. There will be few people. I think only twelve. Don't let the priest take advantage of you, I already paid him for the service. Just ask him to stay for a meal."

I made mental note of all of this, not doubting that it would happen when and as she explained. I had a front row seat to a miracle and ventured to ask with a sizeable lump of tears in my throat, "Can you see the other side? What can you tell me about it? Do you now know the secret of life?" feeling slightly stupid for it all.

Daria was silent for a long while as I both kicked myself for being so naïve to think she would respond and nervously waited to hear what she had to say. I almost gave up.

"I know the secret of life," she said, and then there was a long pause. "You solve one problem and there will be another one to solve. You do it. You just do."

I suppose summarizing all of mankind's deepest conundrums tuckered her out. She closed her eyes and lay back. "One more thing, Lydia. I forgive you for the surgery." And she returned to her coma.

I didn't believe for an instant she could survive another day or two without nutrition or water. But I must admit I was deeply shaken by experiencing her conversing with me, her and her green eyes.

On the morning of June 21, 1986, the nurses urged me to take a break from my daily vigil. I went to the gym. I had sat at my mother's bedside with a stiffened back and knees, for day after day waiting for her to die. I needed a break. I was gone about two hours. I passed the nurses' station on my way back to her room. "No news." I took up my familiar seat on my mother's left side and quietly held her hand. She sneezed. Once. Twice. Then again. And the breath left her.

All my life my parents "kept the cupboards full." I wanted for nothing material. Whatever form the relationship took, after the loss of one parent, I always had my mother as my back-up. With her death I was a full orphan. I was now responsible for filling my own cupboards.

87

Lydia Winslow

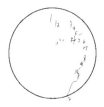

Hot and Bothered

S outh Florida, was a geriatric land of plenty for anyone in the rehab industry. At the Manhattan VA and at Burke, I counted among my patients McKluskys, Cannons, and Magleones. In Miami I treated Solomons, Goldmeiers, and Schmidts, and then in time Gonzalezes, Perezes and Riveras.

Relocating from the New York metropolitan area to South Florida was not such a change in attitude as it was in latitude: after all, some call Miami the sixth borough of New York after Manhattan, Brooklyn, The Bronx, Queens and Staten Island. There were differences: in Manhattan one had the dichotomy of masses of people and individual caring, of face-the-door-don't-talk elevator rides, and the genuine hardy acceptance of neighbors in a neighborhood bar, of grimy well-used streets and walking, shopping and visiting on those streets. In South Florida, one was cool if one did not engage. Snooty was the rule. Your neighbors lived—not on front stoops—but behind their houses on their patios near the pool, and went to work or to the mall in their cars with deeply tinted windows. Many lived in walled-off, gated, nouveau ghetto condos where guests were made welcome by parking in the yellow-curbed guest parking slots miles away from the front door. When you finally reached the front doors, the doormen scrutinized face, manner of dress, and props held while they announced your arrival by phone.

Where else would one step into an elevator and have a very tanned, wizened, short stranger inquire, "So you're here to see Irma? So how is she? Oy, she was so verklempt last night!" Florida! The land of condo commanders, palm cards on Election Day (on which were written the names of the candidates the president of the condo board decided should win), Joe's Stone Crabs and Coppertone.

Where else could you shop for food with French Canadian "snowbirds" in Speedo bathing suits and bikinis?

88

And, oh yes, unremitting heat and humidity.

I worked for a woman named Stephanie who, over the years, had established a solid reputation in the Speech Pathology field through a network of contacts and contracts with the majority of providers in Dade and Broward counties. She, in turn, farmed out hospitals and home health positions to a collection of SLPs, and I primarily worked with home health and with several hospital contracts. Stephanie provided me with a client's name, their address, diagnosis, and the doctor's name. I, in turn, provided her with half my paycheck. Actually my Florida salary surpassed what I made in Manhattan or Westchester—a big and happy surprise.

In Manhattan, I had worked at the VA and noticed my patients had few visitors. Even prior to 9/11, getting into federal buildings like the VA was difficult. When one did gain access, there were set visiting hours allowing patients to get treatment without families tripping over therapists, doctors, and nurses doing their respective jobs. In South Florida, hospitals had set visiting hours and one or two discreet, uncomfortable visitors would shuffle from foot to foot still holding cellophane wrapped bouquets, waiting for the moment they could leave.

Home health was truly the window into the intimate habits of people. Home health put me into people's homes, and therefore, into their lives. I treated an elderly woman—Mrs. F—who had lived with her son in a smallish apartment. The apartment was in a building on South Beach that looked like something on a Hollywood movie set. You climbed two steps into a courtyard tiled in multicolored ceramic. The building pretended to be something out of Arabian Nights. Walk through one of three ornate arches, climb up one flight, and you are in a narrow hallway the likes of which you'd probably see in the Casbah. Knock on an oversized wooden plank door and wait for Mrs. F's flamboyantly attired son to let you in. The also flamboyantly attired designer, Versace, eventually bought the building, and then was murdered on the street in front of it. It is now a fancy South Beach hotel catering to the rich and famous. I look at it and still see Mrs. F. and her doting son in their tiny apartment. That second floor window on the left.

My patients' homes came in all sizes, locations and décor. Some of my patients had views of a back alley's garbage and some had views of the ocean. My population was mainly Jewish, many who were tattooed concentration camp survivors. I became used to being asked if I was Jewish, followed by a frown and a pitying shake of the head when I said no. I assumed my Jewish patients were seeking a deep connection or they did not trust not-Jews. When my patients started making progress, I started looking pretty good and eventually became accepted.

Of course, Miami was made up of many cultures, the majority of which were divided into three groups: whites, either native Floridians or imports from the north; blacks, either Southerners or Jamaicans or Haitians; and Hispanics, mostly Cubans. These cultures did not get along very well, and the Miami Herald told stories of clashes among the groups. In New York, crime was fairly sensible: someone had what someone else wanted and was either shot, stabbed, raped, or mugged and left bleeding on the street. In South Florida crime leaned toward the psychedelic: murders were senseless, random and many times exotic. One very quickly got the impression that every canal in a peninsula crisscrossed with canals was filled and ready to burst with moldering corpses.

Remarkable news coverage included a Hispanic man sitting under a highway overpass, against the concrete holding his dead wife's head in his lap. Another story told of a Midwestern couple on their first trip to Florida. Their hotel room had an unpleasant odor, which, by the second day, was too much to be ignored. The couple reported the smell to the front desk, and a bored hotel employee eventually came up to their room to investigate; a corpse was found under the mattress in the platform bed. You can't make this stuff up.

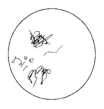

Gracie

In a small, stucco house on a cul-de-sac of a tree-lined street of modest stucco houses lived a single mom, her son, two dogs, and Grace. An attractive petite woman named Cris answered my knock at the door, accompanied by two Great Danes, one black and white, and one brindle. Coming in the side door, I noted a decided lack of furniture but two futon couches, one for each dog, apparently, because each dog stepped onto its own futon and curled up. I had never before seen couches specifically made for pets. Cris said it kept the dogs off the people furniture, which I suspected was in another part of the house.

I asked Cris for background on her mother, my patient. My input sheet was very brief: only that Grace B. had had a stroke, maybe two. She was bedbound, had aphasia, right-sided weakness, diabetes, high blood pressure, and other medical issues. Her background included her address, date of birth, doctor's name and one line that said only "history of psychosis."

History of psychosis, huh? This might be interesting, I mused.

"Okay," I told Cris, "I'm ready to meet your mom."

Grace was lying in a small bedroom and craned her neck to see who was entering. She was propped up in her hospital bed, which overwhelmed the room. The metal railing of the bed on the right was up against an ancient wooden dresser stacked with medical supplies. The bed itself was kitty-corner in the room so that one had to sidle around the left side to a narrow triangular aisle. Grace had a TV in front of her on a mismatched bedside table. It was turned on and probably stayed on all day for noise or to keep Grace company. Cris flicked the TV off. She managed to squeeze a kitchen chair into the room so I could sit close to Grace, and then she left me alone with her.

I sized Grace up. It's strange to say, but the first thing I noticed was the brightly patterned mismatched linens covering her. Grace's head, neck, and shoulders were visible, and her short salt-and-pepper gray hair was cow-licked in different directions. She had a rubbery expressive face, a massive ear-to-ear toothless grin, and the craziest pair of eyes I had ever seen. When not squeezed shut by her cheek-expanding smile, one eye looked east and the other north. The goofy expression on her face didn't quite match up to meeting a stranger and therapist for the first time. I chalked this discordance up to the psych history notation that was on her information sheet.

Curious, I thought.

Grace was friendly enough. She smiled constantly, displaying a lack of most of her natural teeth. She didn't speak and when I spoke to her, she did not peer at me the way some individuals do when they don't understand what is being said. Grace just stared in two different directions and grinned.

I introduced myself and asked her what her name was. After a long, long pause, she said something that sounded like "Grooof." Her voice was hoarse in quality, low, and gravelly. Speaking required much effort and she took her time. I suspected some muscle weakness due to her stroke, because of her speech and because speaking only happened on one side of her face. I routinely performed the parts of the evaluation I needed in order to have enough information for a preliminary report that would provide me reason to return.

Two days later I was prepared with a central goal: "To maximize residual expressive and receptive communication skills to allow the patient to participate in her own management in the home." This was a favorite all-purpose goal I made up for myself which fit all occasions, like a good Hallmark card. It was simply written, but vague enough to include all possibilities. Under this larger goal were assorted short term goals and time frames such as: "This patient will reliably answer simple questions requiring a 'yes' or 'no' response in eight of ten trials in first three weeks," or "This patient will count to ten independently one-hundred percent of the time after three consecutive sessions," and similar items. I had diagnosed Grace as having "markedly severe expressive language deficit combined with moderately slurred speech intelligibility, markedly severe dysphonia, and relatively spared mild to moderate receptive skills." The thrust of my therapy with this patient was creative stimulation of whatever communication skills the stroke left her as well

92

as strategies she and her family could use to fill in for what was perhaps permanently erased.

Sometimes the easiest route to accessing what a person needs is asking for a "yes" or "no" response—a head gesture, pointing to the words or saying the words. Some impacted patients successfully use a communication board and point to pictures of activities, or to large, bold alphabets to spell what they want. Grace left me the impression that her stroke (or strokes) left her with scant ability to get across "bathroom," "hungry," "wet," "never mind" "Trade half of my AT&T for 200 blocks of an overseas growth fund."

I worked painstakingly with Grace on the basics: counting, reciting days, saying her name—easy things that would give her some reward but would not be too taxing. I saw her requiring long-term help merely to provide responses to very simple questions. I doubted she would ever start a request or put more than two or three words together to form a sentence. Socially, Grace was as I described—kind of goofy.

I had been working with Grace three times a week for about one month and it was always the same: Cris opened the door, the Danes escorted me to Grace's door, and I visited with Grace alone. The Danes then dropped lazily onto their respective couches. I never saw Grace out of bed. Cris had said her mother was totally dependent upon her for everything.

Grace seemed to like our time together; she wouldn't take one or both of her eyes off me, and always had an attitude of positive expectation.

My visits started routinely enough: Cris, dogs, alone with Grace. Take materials out of bag, get out my pencil and notebook. I was, I had to admit, getting very bored with the routine and the slow, prodding progress that Grace was making. But Grace never seemed tired of our routine. It was an effort for her to respond but she grinned throughout.

We went over her numbers, "1-2-3, 3 ah, 4-5-7, ah 6…" and her unfinished short sentences "I see with my…eyes," "I shampoo my…hair"…and her name.

This time a tiny, sweet voice responded, "Gracie."

The rhythm of the session was broken by the unfamiliar sounding voice: decidedly not hoarse and definitely not slurred.

"Who are you?" I asked.

"My name is Gracie." This voice was sing-songy, high-pitched and clear in quality.

"How old are you?" I ventured.

"I'm six," she replied. The eyes still held my gaze, but now they were wide open and somehow more childlike. Grace's big, round eyes crinkled almost shut when she grinned.

She sat straighter in her hospital bed and I decided to proceed with my reality orientation assessment. Holding my breath, I asked her where Grace was.

"She's in here with the others."

What others? Again, I asked what her name was.

"Gracie."

"And how old are you?"

"I'm six."

"I told you not to talk to her!" a clear, deeper pitched voice scolded.

My patient started to whimper just like a child. I thought about how strange this was. The session was over as far as Grace (Gracie) was concerned. Her eyes closed and she appeared to be asleep.

On my way out, I corralled Cris. "Tell me more about your mom. When you said your mom was strange, what did you mean? There is a notation on her home health record that just says 'psychiatric.' Did anyone give her a formal diagnosis?"

She asked only, "What happened?"

I told her that maybe it was my imagination, but I thought that there were two different people in that room just now.

After a pause and a deep surrendering exhalation, Cris responded, "She trusts you." She went on, "It isn't schizophrenia, it's something else. It feels like it's something else. She talks to herself, sure, but she...changes, her voice changes."

"Was it always like this?" I asked.

"Yes. What a trip my childhood was. I was raised by my mother, my aunt, a little kid and God knows how many other people. All *in* her!"

"Who else is there?"

"A man, I think…"

"Who else has heard her, does she let the others out?" I asked.

"No one," Cris said, "Mom is very careful, she trusts you."

Later at home, I recalled *Sybil*, the movie, and of course *The Three Faces of Eve*. These were cinemagraphic portraits of something called multiple personalities. Different than schizophrenia, which, as I understand, is a psychotic departure from general reality, accompanied by auditory and or visual hallucinations, and the classic "voices" one hears commanding the individual to do something. Multiple personality syndrome, however, is not strictly a psychosis. The person is functional in society until and unless one or more of the personalities prevent the dominant personality, the one shown to the outside world, from experiencing events. The person may report black outs, memory loss, or confusion. Multiple personality disorder is thought to be caused by the fragmenting of ego in order for the psyche to tolerate unspeakable horror such as sexual or physical abuse in childhood. It is a coping mechanism, a way to bury or catalog intolerable events in order to survive. Until disintegration takes place, for whatever reason, the personalities either don't know about each other or maintain strict control within so that, to the outside world, the multiple appears not unusual.

I documented briefly what I needed to about that session for Medicare and I wrote down the interesting stuff for myself. I was to treat Grace's communication problem arising from her stroke; listing her "extra" symptoms was not within my professional scope. This would stay among Cris, myself and the Gracies.

Visiting the Gracies became a treat. No longer bored, I looked forward to the simple tasks of repeated numbers, the basic orientation questions and the completed sentences. I wanted to see how many people I could tease out. Gracie freely told me, in clear, childlike, pitched voice and, amazingly, in fluid sentences, that she was six, that her mother was very, very strict and didn't like her to speak. Gracie did not appear to be as frightened of her mother whose gruff voice I sometimes heard as the young Grace who was about thirteen-to-fifteen years of age. Young

Grace seldom came out.

I then met a toddler whose speech was barely intelligible. "And what's your name, little girl?" I asked. "No one gave me a name. I have no name." With lurching heart, I sensed this was the core personality—the one who hid. A young boy surprised me by making a rather dramatic appearance, which was shocking because he was able to speak to me and he gestured with Grace's paralyzed right arm.

Nah, I thought, *I am making this up. I am making this whole thing up so I'd have something cool to tell my friends.* But no, it was real.

I gaped as the young boy freely clapped his hands in glee and then waved goodbye to me. He held his arm, in fact the whole body, in a posture characteristic of a male adolescent—very different than the feeble bedbound woman I had come to treat. It was real and it happened only once. The hairs on my neck were definitely standing at attention. Holy shit! The two Danes and their matching couches ceased to be the most interesting thing about this patient.

Through the weeks that Grace was assigned to me, I engaged in a wholly creative and exotic communication. I wanted to nail down the characteristics of each personality, and then compare the voices, the gestures, and the affect each one showed to the other. I did this in Grace's small bedroom with the door closed and nobody else there but me, Grace, Gracie, no-name, the little boy, and the mother. Cris never intruded and after my initial interview with her, never showed much interest in which personality of Grace's I was treating. This was old hat to her, a lifelong magical mystery tour.

I contacted high-level professionals that I knew in the fields of neurology and psychology to see if anyone had ever heard of selective paralysis. I approached each with the question, "Could a multiple 'live' in a healthy part of a stroke victim's brain and be unaffected by the stroke?" Most of the experts I spoke with hadn't had exposure to multiple personalities and could only speculate.

Years later, while substituting for my business partner in her nursing home while she was away, I met Grace again. She was seated in a wheelchair. She exhibited a stroke with right sided paralysis. She did not speak much and stared at those around her. She caught my eye. I received a toothless lopsided grin and one of those crazy-looking eyes winked at me.

In hindsight, it was more probable that the paralysis was used—exaggerated perhaps—adopted for whatever reason by a physically intact representative personality. Maybe Grace's paralysis was "put on." I'll never know; there is nothing in the literature that addresses this strange phenomenon.

Dick

The address was one of Broward County's most prestigious, not because it was on the ocean, it wasn't, but because of the size of the acreage: a huge horse ranch in Plantation Acres along the eastern edge of the Everglades. The patient was middle-aged and he had had a stroke.

The trip out to this ranch took me from the ocean, west on six-lane boulevards, two-lane blacktops, and then a gravel road. The house sat far back behind high, double wrought-iron gates topped in big gold letters announcing the ranch's name *Golden Bough*. I guess it could be called a house in some quarters, but castle would be more accurate, turret and all.

I pulled up in the driveway, parked, and approached the super-sized double front doors. Before I knocked, I peered through the beveled glass window in one door and scanned the entryway. It was vast. The response to my ring was a stoop-shaking commotion, and the door was opened by a person, no doubt, but all I saw were four super-sized Rottweilers. My first instinct was to run, but before I could, the huge dogs float-carried-pushed-herded me into the house and deposited me in front of their mistress. I wondered why *all* of my homebound patients did not have giant protective entry dogs!

I was in a high-ceilinged room with a massive, round, rough-hewn wooden table that could seat about fifteen people. On my right were several clusters of cushy sofas and a giant taxidermied grizzly bear posed to look vicious, in front of a two-story hearth. The bear looked positively petite in that cavernous den (no pun). In front of me, glass and more glass gave a view of the castle's backside: two barns, fences, land, and more land, horses, and more horses. But all I could think of were the four Rottweilers now sniffing my behind.

Kate introduced herself and led me into their beautifully appointed industrial-sized kitchen that managed to seem warm and welcoming. Dick sat waiting for me at one end of a long trestle table. I imagined a table like this in King Arthur's kitchen with chunks of roasted beast and goblets of wine. Dick was in his forties, with black hair, and was ruggedly healthy looking—except for his nasty stroke. His paunch told of many good dinners. The belly strained against an expensive silk guayabara shirt exotically patterned with palm trees and a blue ocean. Dick had poise and a commanding, superior presence, a man used to ordering others around. Now he sat quietly and examined me.

I went through my preliminaries. Dick's response to me was to rise, take my hand, and lead me into his garage. What was this? Waving his hand over his shiny new silver Maserati convertible and using barely understood speech, he basically challenged, "Fix me, you get the car." I laughed and retorted, "I don't want your car, sir, but I wouldn't mind one of your dogs."

When we returned to the kitchen and began our evaluation session, I was keenly aware of his unmistakable thick German accent. As Dick struggled to respond to my very basic questions, his wife Kate stood nearby shaking her head. I couldn't ignore her any longer. "What?" I asked.

"I wanna know where the accent came from."

I punted, "Sometimes when a person has a stroke, he returns to his first, his native language. It's easier, I guess. Not unusual."

"Yeah, I understand. But Dick's not German. Not even close. His native language is Brooklyn."

Okay, that was weird. I took Dick through the usual formal test items and listened extra carefully to him while he spoke. Nope, it was definitely German. He sounded as if had just gotten off the plane from Frankfurt.

He couldn't be faking it, could he? I mean, why would he?

Twenty years later, talk shows will introduce us to a woman who was not remotely Irish but after getting hit on the head, spoke with a thick Irish brogue. And to a man who spoke in what sounded like French. I didn't know enough at this time, in the '80s, to think much about this.

Dick was a man who appeared hale and hearty, a middle-aged bon vivant who loved luxurious cars and thoroughbred horses. Like his horses, his personality was larger than life. His body held a secret: years of gourmandizing and illicit drug enjoyment created a lousy circulatory system, a heart ready to explode, and a brain devastated by stroke. But golly, he looked marvelous.

For weeks Dick teased me with that damn Maserati. "Fix me and the car is yours!"

I wouldn't have refused that car, but always reminded him that he could reward his good little speech therapist with a Rottie.

Visiting Dick and Kate was second to going to Disney World. They toured me through their home: they had a hot tub in a vast two-story stone cylindrical turret room, his and hers black-tiled bathrooms—his with a room-sized shower, hers with a bidet. The hallway into their master suite alone was so large it could have accommodated my entire house. Their horse ranch specialized in stud services. And girls, you ain't lived until you see *that* in living color up close and personal. *Oh my!* One day after a therapy session with Dick, Kate led me back to the barn to witness the birth of a colt.

On the home front, my best friend, my long-time mutt Alex, was dying. He had reached the tender age of sixteen and had been by my side from the moment I found him tied to a playground fence in the West Village; he lived with me under my one-bedroom apartment's bed, and then to Florida in his final home in the Hollywood Hills, where we had met our neighbors through the graces of the police SWAT team. Years later, Alex-dog tenderly guarded my newborn baby boy when we brought Ian home from the hospital. When I woke up every two hours to nurse, my best friend Alex woke up too, and trailed out to the living room to lay next to me and my child all through the night. But Alex was losing weight; my new motherhood could not distract me away from noticing. Eventually, Alex stopped eating altogether and lay at my feet. He died shortly afterward.

I had Dick on my schedule the next day and wanted to call and cancel. But I went. I blew through a stop sign on my way to his home and saw blue lights behind me. When the officer came to my window, I was in full-blown sorrow. The stress of losing my dog and now getting stopped by a cop just put me over the edge. "I'm so sorry officer," I blubbered, "My dog died." The officer let me go. I mourned mightily. I loved that dog like no other. He was the closest thing to me when I needed him the most, in my many transitions, through a lot of years. My reddened nose and wet eyes were immediately noticed. Kate and Dick were dog lovers, dog breeders, animal whisperers. They flanked me and comforted me.

Dick's communication improved gradually. As his German persona faded, more Brooklyn peeked out, and I took this as a sign that he was resuming normalcy. He still had peculiar word-finding substitutions and stammered in his efforts to speak. When the hausenfrauemnier morphed into goddamn somabitch, Kate pronounced Dick back to normal.

As my time with Dick came to an end and I made plans to discharge him from service, Kate and Dick sat me down and announced, "Our stud Rottie's mate just had her pups and we are giving you pick of the litter."

I thought to myself, *What about the damn car?*

I was, of course, moved and very grateful for their gesture of thanks; further because I knew the depth of their gift. Their male's father was a recognized award winner, his picture gracing the cover of the AKC standards manual for Rottweilers. The female belonged to a breeder who Dick trusted. We made a date to visit the pups. I picked out a sweet, gorgeous female and marked her with a pink collar. I could come get her when she was old enough to leave her mother. My heart sang. I shopped the pet stores for all things girly-dog, things I'd need to welcome her home. Alex left a huge hole to fill, and my new dog would be very loved.

After I brought my new pup home, Kate and Dick asked me what her name was; her AKC title name as well as her everyday name. The everyday name was a no-brainer. I named her Dixie so she'd remember her godfather, Dick. Dixie was beautiful and so very sweet. She went willingly to obedience school at six months and learned quickly all the doggie stuff they taught. She loved us so much. Hearts flew out of my head whenever I looked at her.

We would bring her to a watering hole and she would doggie-paddle around with my four-year-old hugging her neck. She swam with my son around and around without complaint. Dixie took to heeling quickly and walked docilely through the neighborhood with each of us.

One high-pitched cry when she was about ten months old alerted me to a potential problem, but she looked okay and didn't cry out again. Soon after, while on a walk, she plopped down on the sidewalk and looked up with evident pain in her eyes. I took her to our vet with a heavy heart. The X-ray revealed minimal development of a hip socket, common dysplasia in my pick-of-the-litter pup. The stress of the pain in her hip also caused skin problems, which were not easily addressed. My baby Dixie went from a sweet and good-natured pup to a sweet, good-natured sick pup. The vet suggested putting her down.

I held out for several weeks hoping for a recovery of some sort. A phone call from Kate let me know that Dick had suffered a major heart attack. He did not survive. Kate was, of course, tearful but resolute that she could handle the ranch herself. "Come see me," she requested.

Across the familiar trestle table over coffee, I asked Kate what to do about Dixie. "I don't want to lose her."

"Something went wrong with the litter. Many of these pups had the same sort of skin issues you're telling about and one had to be put down. Don't let little Dixie suffer. Let the vet put her down."

Both of us stared moodily into our coffee mugs glad for each other's company and sad to the core.

Dixie taught me a hard lesson: Don't name a pup after a very sick patient.

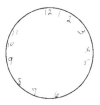

Chastity

Picture the stereotypical witch in a children's theatre production: brittle gray-and-white hair uncombed standing straight out kind of like photographs of Einstein. A pre-Colombian shrunken head covered in pale Shar Pei wrinkles. A rubber mouth opening impossibly wide to show off one or two determined teeth. Now imagine this creature's eyes. No I don't think you can. The eyes are alive, compelling, they hold you and invite you. So now the reader can picture Chastity. But that's not the whole tale.

Chastity had been diagnosed with amyotrophic lateral sclerosis nearly four years before she had become my patient. This is unusual given that victims of Lou Gehrig's disease seldom make it beyond two years with the notable exception of Stephen Hawking, now having survived decades with the disease. At the time of Chastity, I had already counted two very memorable ALS victims among my patients. I knew little more than it was a death sentence and an ugly one. Typically, the ALS victim is in late middle age. The first complaint may be overall weakness and fatigue or more likely difficulty getting a lungful of air. The devastation races rapidly to the muscles of the tongue, disabling swallow and speech. It may attack one side of the body over the other but without being able to take in food by mouth and feeling weakened, that "*laterality*" of ALS is a nonissue. The muscles of the shoulder blades and thumb to index finger pads become hollowed. The scapulae stick out like wings. This hollowing is a result of muscles *atrophying*. ALS is a progressive neurodegenerative disease of the brain and spinal cord. As the disease progresses, the nerves within the area affected harden or become "*sclerosed.*" Hence the label to this nightmare: a myotrophic – lateral – sclerosis.

That cute, three-letter acronym doesn't begin to describe the nightmare of ALS: while the body wastes away, the mind stays alive and watches. It's brain damage in a very special sense. The voice and speech of an ALS is unmistakable—that is, before the voice and speech disappear altogether. With little breath support and a tongue that barely moves, the person sounds monstrous, kind of like Darth Vader with asthma. One desperate word at a time…pains…takingly…doled…out…

Chastity was bedbound, tended to by her husband. Looking at her, one could get the feeling that her barely mobile hands and compelling eyes were the only living parts that remained of the woman called Chastity. I was a latecomer to Chastity: much of the damage of ALS had already been done.

Chastity was fed soupy puree, foods that were blended and then thinned down to the consistency of gruel, with liquids thickened to the consistency of honey. Her spouse placed each spoonful into her open lips and Chastity had to tip back her head to allow the food to fall into her throat. Her tongue had given up the fight and just laid there.

Chastity hadn't surrendered verbal communication. She bellowed out gusts of wind with an undercurrent of noise, but it wasn't speech anymore. Nevertheless, she "talked." She would get a word out edgewise and that's what it sounded like. I pondered what I could do to help her.

Chastity and her husband lived in a smallish duplex in the definition of a single-story building with two adjacent dwellings. If you walked in the front door—whap!—there she was, right inside the door in her hospital bed that didn't fit anywhere else in the place.

I sidled around the bed and pulled up the aluminum folding chair that her husband had ready for me. Chastity opened her mouth and laughter exploded into the room. Her shoulders trembled, her eyes squinted and gusts of air filled the room. It was Chastity-style laughter. I wondered if Chastity in her younger, pre-ALS days was one of those girls that giggled to punctuate. Chastity looked the crone of children's theater but she was only forty-eight.

I didn't waste too much time agonizing over how to treat Chastity. It was clear that she was incapable of articulating her words and was fairly content with how she could manage her food. But she kept talking to me. She had lots of things to say. I had a thought: Since she had some lingering use of her hands and fingers, I would enhance her ability to communicate by working on her writing. It was a worthwhile thought, but it wasn't very effective. Chastity had difficulty grasping a pen, a pencil, or fat crayon. I proposed that her husband buy her a computer. She frowned at this idea. Her husband rejected buying a computer. They had much better places to put their dwindling savings, like into medical care. Instead I went to an office supply store for information and got the name of a repairman who still sold old electric typewriters. I paid him twenty dollars for a mint-condition IBM Selectric and carried it to Chastity's.

She didn't need lessons; she had as much experience with typewriters as I once had in those days before iPads and laptops. As I sat patiently, she tapped out, "Thank you for the typewriter. Can you help me with something?" I agreed, thinking she had something basic to communicate: move the TV closer, change the channel, call my husband, give me another blanket.

"Help me die," she typed.

I didn't move, just stared at her. She tapped away, "Give me all of my medication at once."

After collecting myself, I was just as blunt as she had been. "Nope. If you want to die, you are going to have to do it by yourself. I refuse to kill you."

But she insisted, "You won't kill me. Just put the pills on my table and I will take them. I will kill myself."

"No. Doing that will be an action I would have to take. I will not actively kill you. If you want to die, you will have to do it yourself."

"How?" she queried.

So began my strange relationship with Chastity.

Beneath the gusts of laughter and the sparkling eyes, I knew she was dead serious about wishing to end her suffering. But I wasn't playing this game. I was merely patronizing her, and in reality, discouraged her from doing anything that would end her life. Still, with her sense of humor being as black as mine, I was willing to debate her on how a person with very little ability left at her disposal could muster a method to die.

Together we ruled out many scenarios: jump out the window, but that wouldn't work. They lived on the ground floor and she couldn't get to the window. I couldn't get to the window—the hospital bed took up all the room. Gun or knife? Both would need another person to actually work. Poison? Either her husband or I would have to get it and leave it accessible for her. It was the same with her medications. Besides, she had grave difficulty swallowing and would probably throw up.

"Chastity, no one else is going to kill you. You have to kill yourself. And the only way you can actively kill yourself is to stop eating. Starve. That is something you still have control over." As I was putting my things together to leave for the day, she was actually thinking about this.

The following week started with a visit to Chastity. She was still alive and she was still trying to verbalize. She was still open-mouth laughing at whatever. Her eyes indicated I should sit. Her Selectric and a sheaf of papers sat on her hospital tray table. The eyes pointed to the papers. I picked them up and read.

Chastity had spent her weekend, not pondering ways to kill herself, but writing. She had about thirty pages for me to read. It was her journal, as titled, and it was pure porn. Extravagant, delicious, juicy, purple pornography. I asked her what her plans were and she typed for me:

"Book. Thanks for the Selectric. I'll be dead soon enough."

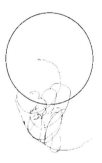

Alchemy

A round the time I met and treated Dick (1984-85), I had a lucrative contract with a hospital in North Miami. During the years I worked there, I shared that facility with two other practices: a North Miami-based single-woman practice which was very well respected, and the original group that the three of us had broken away from years earlier. North Miami Medical Center decided to make my practice their exclusive provider of speech services. It was a great contract. North Miami Medical Center turned out to be the alchemist for the rest of my life.

My administrator at NMMC called me into his office one day. Usually a call to the administrator's office was about doing more work for less money, or scolding me for disagreeing with a physician, and I felt the way I did when called to the principal's office—like a bad little kid. The administrator, Tom F., informed me that he was leaving NMMC to administer a new, free-standing rehabilitation hospital in western Broward County. He asked if I wanted to join him and start South Florida's premier free-standing rehabilitation hospital. It was an exciting prospect and I loved a professional challenge. But I needed to decide what to do about my private practice.

Tom said that the rehab hospital was in planning stages. Ground breaking had not yet happened, so I had time. My responsibilities were to develop equipment needs, meet the other people involved in scheduled planning meetings, and familiarize myself with the requirements of CARF (Commission on the Accreditization of Rehabilitation Facilities). "Besides," he said, "you will probably be able to keep your private contracts since your position as head of the speech department will only be part-time. Speech Therapy will only see about ten percent of the total census."

I accepted the job with Rehabilitation's Optimal Therapies or 'ROT' for short. For about a year I was the department head of a one-person speech department without a building to work in and no patients with whom to work. That year I was paid for the actual hours I put in. When the hospital received its certificate of need and actually opened, I received an annual salary based on the part-time work ROT thought would be necessary. That hospital was more successful than anticipated, and before long, I had to hire three other SLPs and a speech aide. The management kept me on as 'part-time' even though the people who worked for me were all full time. I patiently waited for them to change my employment status and issue a check for retroactive salary differential. It was only a matter of paperwork, right?

My two-year old son at this time was in the care of a nanny. Having the support I needed on the home front, I dove into the work of organizing a department with gusto.

I had been working on my own for most of my career. I didn't have a clear picture where on the medical totem pole the speech pathologist's profile was carved. When I contract with a facility—inpatient or outpatient—I come in, do my job, and then leave. At ROT, the physical therapy director huddled with the occupational therapy director huddled with the clinical supervisor. I was not included in the major decisions. At the very least they could have bought me a chew toy.

Given the responsibility and the education we as a large group have, it didn't seem to me that we were held in high regard. I am freely using the first person plural here because this has been what I've observed and heard from my colleagues in different medical settings. This has been one of my biggest disappointments. In the public schools, speech language pathologists are considered separate—not better, not worse—but separate, from classroom teachers. Speech language pathologists are under the special education label. We are all certified by ASHA, and in most states, hold licenses to practice speech language pathology in addition to a teacher's certification. School therapists typically have two to five children at a time. At times there is friction between the classroom teachers with thirty children and the SLPs. The classroom teachers resent the SLP taking their (their!) kids out of class for treatment.

In medicine, the SLP gets orders to evaluate and treat from a physician. Many doctors simply don't put a premium on communication. Their priority, naturally, is getting the body well. Nurses throughout my career have verbalized that they could do my job, both the swallowing and the communication. They challenge, "You only see them once a day for an hour, who do you think takes care of these people the rest of the time?" Besides, the work of the PT and the OT are visible: They walk their patients. They help dress their patients. They transfer their patients from bed to chair and back.

I felt and still feel that as a profession, speech-language pathologists are under-utilized. We don't have the top billing that physical therapists do. There's a good argument that PTs are generally better paid and busier in some settings because more disability groups are seen by PTs than SLPs. SLPs don't, typically, treat orthopedic patients—as an example, unless the patient has a communication, cognitive, or swallowing problem. I'm grumbling, maybe because I didn't want to be 'behind the scenes' anymore.

I believe that many of my fellow SLPs are satisfied and comfortable in their own skin as I seldom was. Many of the SLP's I was encountering didn't challenge themselves. They didn't take advantage of the opportunities for intensive and divergent training available to us by ASHA. The majority of my profession is trained to correct children's articulation. The SLP going into the medical or academic fields had to step off the track and get education in whatever subfield the SLP might be interested in. I have met many colleagues who agree to work with neurologically impaired patients but absolutely would not go near a tracheostomy. Others work with phonation and don't own a ten-foot pole with which to touch an autistic. For many years, the SLP had the highest education level compared to PTs and occupational therapists in the medical arena. Of all three professions, aside from a doctor's order to evaluate and treat, the SLP did not need the doctor to specify what type of treatments to perform—as was the case with PTs and OTs. The SLP determines if the patient requires swallowing rehabilitation, language treatment, or oral motor work—how much and how long. With the responsibility of treating a fragile population, which included those with aspiration pneumonia, I assumed SLPs would be given more respect. Not at that time, not at that rehab hospital. Not me.

I didn't have star billing. I was running a department that was behind physical therapy *and* occupational therapy in terms of *anticipated* utilization (translation, generation of income), *and I was part-time.* I became the biggest chump on the planet when I, driven to prove myself as an SLP, as an originator of a brand new department (and a darned good person), worked at that rehab hospital more than four hours a day, often more than eight hours a day. And for practically no pay. I confess that patching together an entire department in a brand new facility was exciting and fun. I suppose that's what kept me there. However, those first days after the hospital opened its doors had kept me at work long after dark, stressed and despondent that my little boy was growing up without me.

I needed to wake up and smell the writing on the wall.

I again reminded my supervisor, who reported to Tom F., that I was waiting for my change of status to full-time with a raise in pay from part-time to full-time. I asked—and this time, was refused. He told me, "There's no great need for speech. You should have been a PT. They have to see everyone in the hospital. Besides, the budget won't allow it," he'd said.

Then, one day when I was doing some department work on pay stubs, I just happened to see the human relations department files. A starting Physical Therapy *assistant's* salary at ROT was higher than my "part-time" salary as a *department head* in which I had been putting in ten hours a day, with a staff of four. *Salt in the wound.* But I stayed. I was undervalued—but I stayed. Being undervalued was an early-learned trait of mine. As was my habit, I turned my rage inward. I did and said stupid things to those in charge. I didn't know enough to leave. I wasn't brave enough to negotiate and bargain myself a better deal. Asserting myself just did not occur to me. Lessons I thought I had learned early in my career in the world-class rehabilitation center in Westchester, New York apparently were forgotten.

A month after the space shuttle *Challenger* exploded, so did I. I think the day I told my supervisor (in writing, copying his superiors) what a total asswipe he was, was when everyone—including Lydia—decided it was time for Lydia to go. So the parting was mutual. Things were becoming untenable for me at ROT, and the important work of getting accredited and forging a department was done. The hospital had met CARF Accreditization and the day-to-day labor had begun. And, I was grossly miserable. And because I was grossly miserable, I made everyone around me equally miserable. I didn't wish to remain there and my supervisor didn't want me to remain there.

Perhaps in another industry, my employers would have valued me and would have fought for me to stay and be happy. I would have been seen as valuable. I would have been offered perks and incentives. Perhaps in another industry my skill set would off-set my temperament. Once more, I questioned if this field was a good fit for me.

I returned to business-as-usual with my private practice, my beautiful resilient private practice, kept afloat by my two dear partners and several impressively accommodating clients. The practice that grew out of three ambitious women who had needed to go it alone, Petty, Schrager and Winslow, P.A., was successful. But in 1988, ten years after the Professional Association was incorporated, we decided that a corporate structure no longer worked to our advantage and the three of us dissolved. I started my own practice, Lydia Winslow, M.A. and Associates, and after we divvied out the existing contracts, I still had a lucrative and successful practice.

The same year that saw the breakup of Petty, Schrager & Winslow, P.A. saw the breakup of my marriage. Both began in January of 1978 and both ended in 1988. Coincidence? My husband had moved out, but not far away from me and our five-year-old son, Ian. The way I saw it, we had a civilized, mature, co-parenting arrangement. No, that's a lie. I believe, and I think Art would years later agree, that our separation and subsequent divorce was ugly, childish, petty, and violent. But I don't wish to relive that in these pages. I felt the same undisguised contempt from my husband that I felt from my father. It was familiar ground and so it was comfortable for a while. That time in my life just before my separation from Art was a cyclone in a narrow canyon. Gale-force emotional winds buffeted me this way and that, and threatened to slam me into the stone walls of the situation I was in. I would be lifted above to float for a while, oblivious to danger, and for a breath, at peace.

I was flying solo this time without a plane around me. Although in a vortex of shifting emotions, I loved my freedom from all three of my partners: professional and spousal. I could make professional decisions for myself. With shared custody and every other weekend to myself, I could go out and line dance, something I had always loved but husband did not. I had the money to refurbish and redecorate my house any damn way I wanted. And no dirty socks on the floor.

I had about a year more of solid work at North Miami Medical Center before that hospital announced it was to merge into another area hospital and close.

There I was, first to arrive at the goodbye party for the rehab department at North Miami Medical at Bennigan's Restaurant. A colleague, Mary, joined me and we sat in the bar area to await the others. I had been newly single for about a year and two months before my divorce was final. And suddenly, there *he* was. I recognized him instantly, this man I had never seen before. I turned to Mary and announced with utter certainty, "There is my perfect mate." It was a thought. Just a thought. I wasn't tempted to act on it. It was just certitude. Besides, the rest of our party had arrived and we were all seated, our dinners had arrived soon thereafter, and our drinks came and came and came. An hour-and-a-half into our separation party found some of us maudlin over loss of jobs, loss of friends, and the rest of us were drunk and getting seriously silly.

My side of the table was debating whether the size of a man's thumb corresponded to the size of his penis. Mary interrupted by asking me what I proposed to do about my "perfect mate" who was still there at the bar. Nothing. I proposed to do nothing. Mary dared me to invite him to our table. I stood in the middle of a horde of drunken colleagues who were chanting, "Invite him, invite him!" Mary escorted me in case I tried to bolt. To my amazement (and to his own surprise, he later confessed) my "perfect mate" joined my crazy beloved colleagues at our goodbye table.

My perfect mate lived up to his name. Skip Wilkenson became my second husband exactly one year later. Reader, please take note: his name starts with 's.' My oracle, Vincent, told me it would be this way.

I then made another change in my life. With NMMC closing, I decided to get a second master's degree in business administration. I applied and was accepted into the business school of Florida International University and became, yet again, a student.

Ode to a Role Model

"You can draw shoes!" was the first thing Bree had said to me. We shared a patient that first year I worked in Miami and I had left him hand-drawn pictures to name. We both worked for Stephanie and I had met the other two women who stopped in at the Lincoln Road office to grab patient assignments and run. I would have to wait several weeks before meeting Bree Schrager, my future business partner, in person. We had already established a close relationship on the phone. I could draw shoes well—and that was probably the only thing I could do better than Bree.

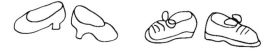

One year later Bree, Nora-with-the-blue-Honda, and I, became business partners. A more divergent threesome could not be found. The petite Romanian Jewess, the tall red-haired Russian, and the Southern belle—or as we were better known in those days, Petty, Schrager, and Winslow, P.A., fine purveyors of excellent speech pathology services in two counties from 1978 to 1988. Despite our differences, we became and have stayed close friends.

I used Bree as my professional encyclopedia. She was ten-plus years ahead of me in the field. She usually gave good advice and was willing to brainstorm to solve a problem. Some of her solutions didn't always work, such as the time she was teaching a head trauma patient who couldn't find the words he had lost, how to gesture when he needed to use the urinal. She quickly realized she was not understood. He couldn't make the connection between pointing to his pants and needing to go to the bathroom. So, Bree clarified this for him by reaching over and grabbing his penis—just as his doctor entered.

For all of her confidence on the job, Bree had a timid side. In the '70s, a master's degree was common among medically based Certified Speech and Language Pathologists. Later a master's degree in the field would be a requirement. Bree had gotten her education and certification before this requirement so she was grandfathered in with only a bachelor's degree. Not having a master's degree apparently bothered her, so Bree decided to go back to school. There were no speech programs offered at that time in the area. Completing a master's in Speech Pathology would have been redundant for Bree—she could have taught the courses, she knew more than most people about the field. Nova University (later Nova Southeastern University) had a master's program

113

in geriatrics, which sounded good to her but, as a middle aged student, she didn't want to go alone. I volunteered to go with her for the first few classes, and I audited several classes myself so she could get started on her degree. I liked that she needed me.

Bree's learning never stopped. She kept up with all the Medicare and insurance regulations and could quote scripture and verse on Federal policy. We had a shared fantasy. We would be Doctors. She and I were going to enroll at the University of Miami's medical school together and split the M.D. we both wanted—she'd be the "M" and I'd be the "D" since that's all the initial we each had time for.

Bree was consulted by hospitals on treatment of the head-injured for the knowledge she had acquired. One could not find a stronger patient advocate. She did daily battle with the nuns, the administration, the doctors, and the rest of the staff at Bon Secours-Villa Maria (a hospital and nursing home combination) to do things her own way and created a speech department nonpareil. A goodly percentage of the speech pathologists working in the South Florida area had at one time or another worked for, or with, Bree. A smaller number, perhaps, sat at her feet and credit her with a lot of professional growth. I still do.

Bree told me once that she had consciously tried to compensate for being a short, cute girl by being a tough, stubborn broad of a woman. Under her crust was a person who suffered unspeakable heartache in her personal life. Her seven-year-old son Amos was hit by a drunk driver as he waited in line at an ice cream truck in the neighborhood in 1973. She celebrated a late-in-life pregnancy after his death, but the celebration was cut short when her husband was diagnosed with a brain tumor, and then died. She was left to raise her fatherless daughter and her two sons alone. Bree had always extended herself for family and for her friends.

Not that Bree didn't bore us all silly with her imagined ailments. She told us she had everything wrong with her. A heavy smoker who had tried quitting many times, she ironically insisted that she just couldn't function in allergy season. When Villa Maria did some plaster repair, Bree had to go home for the duration due to her allergies or asthma or something. She called in sick for a sniffle. We goodheartedly teased her about how sick she thought she was.

I answered the phone one day to hear her son Dwight tearfully tell me, "Mom's dead." She was sixty-two. She died in her sleep of a heart-related condition.

I added my stone to the pile of prayer rocks on her gravesite after the funeral and stood looking down at her. "I guess you really were sick," I said to no one. Today, when faced with a difficult professional question, I turn to Bree to give me spiritual guidance. She does! Bree, I will draw you oxfords, loafers, heels, whatever you like.

I owe you, girl.

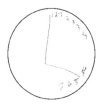

The Girls

Healthcare professionals know the phenomenon of three's: two deaths will bring a third soon. Three charts will have eerily identical diagnoses. There will be three patients of the same nationality with the same types of aphasia. A period in my career when I was in my 30s brought me three young women.

Debbie was twenty-four, Ashley had just turned thirty, and Rosa thirty-six. They all suffered strokes, which impaired only their speech and left their physical movements intact. All were Broca's Aphasics (an expressive disorder with dysfluent speech output with difficulty finding words). All three strokes were related to hormones. Perhaps because of the ages of these women and myself, perhaps because all three were dynamic girls with enough spunk to burn off the effects of their strokes, or maybe all three found something in me to hold onto. Whatever the reason, each has stayed in my life and in my heart forever.

Ashley was a lovely woman of only thirty when her boyfriend brought her to the emergency room when her right hand felt numb. She couldn't speak. She was unable to make sounds and was getting more and more hysterical with the effort. I met her the day after she was admitted. She sat upright in her bed in her cotton blue-printed hospital gown surrounded by her sister, her mom and her boyfriend. I didn't expect someone so young.

When I sat and introduced myself to her and to those who were visiting, she stared at me and performed Lamaze breathing exercises. She blew vigorously into my face over and over, and then sobbed. Her body didn't display that telltale weakness on one side: this slim, pretty girl with long, straight, brown hair, and bangs that brushed her eyes looked half her age. Her history alone told me that she had suffered a major stroke, which had affected her left hemisphere and knocked out all ability to speak. Could she understand me?

I was unsure since she was very emotional and was too distraught to respond effectively. She continued to blow. I was feeling out of my depth: I didn't know how to tackle this situation. So I blew back at her. I imitated what she did. I gradually added voice: "Whooo. Whooo." She stared hard at me, willing herself to vocalize. When she succeeded in a respectable "Whoo" her tears started again. She had success with the immense effort to just say, "Whoo." I continued with this tactic: I molded my blowing into notes and sounds: "Whoo Who? Aaaah. Ooh," until Ashley managed some different sounds of her own. She could vocalize and differentiate her vocalizations. This was a first big step. I snuck a peek at my watch and was surprised that an hour-and-a-half had gone by. I laughed and said, "You must be exhausted! You must feel like you've dug a ditch!" She smiled and nodded. I wrote down in large letters the time I would return and my name, bid the entourage goodbye, and then left.

My unorthodox treatments with Ashley didn't last long. She remained only a few days at the hospital. The hospital had no reason to keep her since she was not paralyzed. She was able to walk and care for herself. Ashley's insurance covered home visits so she could continue the speech therapy she very much needed. I was lucky enough to continue working with her.

Ashley and Phil lived together in a small, unremarkable apartment. As with other home care patients, I met with her at her kitchen table. It was the easiest arrangement sitting across or next to my client. She could see my face and I hers. And since I often accompanied my spoken therapy with writing or drawing, having a table made this more comfortable. I began with Ashley where I had left off at the hospital, with various, basic vocalizations. Phil stood and watched for a while then asked, "So why did this happen? All of a sudden she couldn't speak."

I discovered that most of my patients, young or old, never had their strokes explained to them. In fairness to their doctors, perhaps this was done, but they were not in a good place emotionally or mentally to comprehend, and did not digest the facts provided. I had included a simplistic primer on stroke and the rehabilitation that I would provide with every case.

I drew a very basic brain and marked with "X's" where I knew skills were localized: in the frontal lobe was Broca's Center where motor

117

speech lived, in the temporal lobe was where Wernicke's area handled understanding of speech. The occipital lobe managed vision and the prefrontal lobe managed, well, managing; it was where executive function was thought to be. Memories were stuck every which way in both the right and left hemispheres and in the white and grey matters. I explained stroke as an interruption of the blood flow to the brain, either by clot or by hemorrhagic "drowning." If a major artery was blocked or bleeding, the end result was a massive stroke that could severely impair or kill the victim. If the clot or bleed was in a smaller "branch" or "twig" of the artery, the effect would be less traumatic.

I went on to tell my patient that, in most people, the dominant side of the brain was the left side (I tap my head on the left.) The nerves originating on that side crossed over lower down in the nervous system around the area of the neck and governed the right side of the body. The dominant hemisphere is where symbolic language is thought to be found. This is good design. Most people are right handed so the language-brain communicates more directly with the right hand. But of course, later we found that pieces and parts of language are helter-skelter throughout the brain in both hemispheres.

I told Ashley that her Broca's area or the part of the brain responsible for speech was now disconnected by the stroke from those areas which held the sequencing of word-sounds as well as from where meaning of words was stored. I used a map, illustrating two large cities. "You can't drive down the freeway to get from 'X' to 'Y' anymore. The stroke knocked out the bridge connecting both sides of the highway. So you have a choice: find a detour which is slower; give up and go home— an option many patients take; or work to rebuild the bridge. This new bridge may be on another part of the highway but, in time, it will make the trip more efficient."

Ashley worked like a demon to rebuild that bridge.

Ashley's medical history included the significant notation that she suffered from migraines. Either her gynecologist was not told of her headaches, or did not cross-reference them to the side effects of the birth control pills he prescribed. The migraines plus contraception was likely the trigger for Ashley's stroke.

Much of the work I did with Ashley was teasing out then shaping sounds. I might have used syllables—either words or nonsense—that started with vowels and added a consonant at the end. If she was successful with a particular consonant, say "p," I would tack a "p" word onto the first word. So "uuuuup" would become "uup pie."

"Ouch" would become "ouch tree." "Eat would become "eat too" and so on. The consonant formed a sort of train, pulling out the initial sound of the second word. Reinforcement of the consonant could be done with word lists of the successfully elicited sounds, going back to the first successful "train" if the patient had trouble.

A "t" word list might go like this: too, tea, moe—no, eat—tea, tea, toe…etc." These little trains were added together so that the initial successful sounds ended up pulling whole phrases.

Speech pathologists either start with the weakest link or the strongest. I will take whatever residual skill my patient has and build on it. However, I tend not to stay with the tasks that are easiest. I quickly move on to more challenging tasks and deliberately 'stress' my patient. I tell them, "I will give you more than you need when you use your speech socially. You'll have more confidence."

Sometimes only an indirect method works to capture an elusive sound. I use spitting, horn-blowing, blowing air out with the tongue in a "raspberry," animal noises—any creative thing I can think of to get that one sound. Then I reinforce the sound and work on others.

Much of what I do is restoring confidence. I hope to never in my own life have to experience the loss of my ability to communicate, but each and every one of my patients has told me at some point that whether the communication was lost through stroke, by being on a ventilator, or through cancer surgery, nothing was more devastating to them than the loss of their most human skill—the ability to speak. *The* most important goal we—my patient and I—set is the restoring of confidence. I am up front with them: the stuff we do together over the bedside table or at the kitchen table will be harder than anything they will face in public. It has to be so that they know they can do it. They can do anything. They can be heroes.

Debbie is a great example of heroic. In her mid-twenties, she experienced the tragedy of being pregnant for the full term only to deliver a stillborn baby. In addition, she stroked during delivery. Like Ashley, Debbie did not suffer physical weakness. Rather, she had difficulty finding words to express herself. If there was any silver lining to Debbie's story it was that she recovered quickly and did not need me long.

Two or three years after her hospitalization, Debbie lived in my neighborhood for a while until she married her true love, Scott, bought a house, and moved. She stayed in steady touch with me. Much to my awe, she made me a needlepoint of an infant when my baby was born, which must have cost her a lot emotionally; the needlepoint of a child was made with love by a woman who could not be a mother herself.

She sent me a card every single year for almost thirty years. One card I received said:

Dear Lydia,

How are you and your family? As for us, just fine. Busy always in the store. It's twenty years since you and I worked together (stroke). I always think of you. If it wasn't for you I'd be different.

Happy holidays to all,

Debbie

Fate was not finished with Debbie: in midlife, she developed cancer and is still—hopefully—in remission. I love you, Debbie! You are MY hero!

Speech pathology is, by its nature, a very social field. I enjoy social interchange. I don't seem to be adept at friendly interaction with friends. I am by nature sarcastic and quick-witted. From an early age, I've sought to get attention by being the clown. I'm not always aware that my words have crushed a dear one's feelings. Social interaction with my patients has always been different. I don't know why.

It is exciting to knock on a stranger's door, offer my eyes on theirs, and start the courtship. It's akin to flirtation, and with any hope, a seduction. And really, whether we are talking about finding a mate or finding a lawyer, bargaining for a purchase, meeting a new neighbor or a brand new patient, isn't it all seduction toward a worthwhile relationship? I come to each meeting equipped with my own thoughts, dreams, goals and philosophies. Hopefully, in the process of meeting and becoming familiar, I will learn of the others' thoughts, dreams, goals and philosophies. I look forward to knowing these strangers: valuable stuff not only about the communication status of this special individual, but also insights on his or her thinking and what he or she is made of, what his or her values are, and if this person will make it through the healing process to become whole. In leisurely conversational sharing, I get a personal history and a far more in-depth medical history than the physician with his or her limited amount of time spent on each patient is privy to. After some time for rapport, of bonding, a trust is built. Eventually, I become the repository of secret needs, of nightmares, of autobiographies and of eulogies. With the powerful tool of rapport I become an interpreter as well, and, as only a mother understands her preverbal child, I glimpse meaning in the facial expression and the postures and the grunts of my aphasic patient, that no one else can.

Rosa was a firebrand Latin who stroked while delivering her daughter. Her stroke was similar to Ashley and Debbie's—she could not find words. Rosa's stroke had another result: it changed her personality. While she had always been spunky with personality to spare, Rosa, a professional businesswoman, was known to be poised and gentle with people. Her work challenged her to be direct and assertive but she always handled people tactfully—but not after her stroke. Her husband, Bob, noticed immediately.

As Rosa's speech became more functional, she expressed impatience and was rude when demanding things she wanted. Working so hard for the very words robbed Rosa's verbal output of subtlety. Her hard-won words were blunt and painfully honest. She was easily frustrated. During the rehabilitation, Bob doted on Rosa. He seemed not to be able to do enough for her. The bond that brought the Latin woman and the German man together was being frayed. One day, Rosa told Bob she felt no love for him anymore. She said she had no idea why she married him in the first place. In discussions with Bob, my husband and I reassured him that "it was the stroke talking, she'll get better." Eventually, many months after my therapy sessions with Rosa were concluded, one or the other would visit us with their daughter, now a toddler. Rosa gradually visited less and less often. Bob remained tightly in our circle of friends. We found more in common with Bob than with Rosa. On one of his visits, he said that Rosa had left, moved on.

∽

The eighties connected me with many exceptional people. Not all of my patients suffered brain damage. A lasting friendship was forged with Dolores, a forty-something cancer victim whose larynx was removed. We worked hard to develop—then perfect—her esophageal speech, the use of air swallowed then brought up from the esophagus—a burp, really. With patience and instruction, this burp is held skillfully in the throat. Then as it passes through the mouth, the air is articulated with jaw, lips cheeks and tongue into recognizable speech sounds. Dolores was a master at speaking using esophageal speech. She sounded like a deep-voiced woman, not at all unnatural. Dolores crafted fashionable silk scarf arrangements to disguise the hole in her neck. She was polished and fashionable with a deep Greta Garbo rasp to her "voice." It was awhile before she challenged herself by going out in public and speaking to clerks or tellers or strangers. One of the first topics she verbalized was the rage she felt at having suffered through cancer. After teaching Dolores how to again speak, I sat back and listened. Our speech therapy sessions enabled her to have an appropriate and private audience before she got the courage to speak to strangers.

Marie was the elderly wife of a well-to-do and well-known businessman whose little banking business early in the 1940s became one of the largest bank institutions in Broward County. I visited her in her elegant waterfront home in the Hollywood Lakes area. Healthy and independent all of her eighty years, she had suffered a stroke. We worked with speech and verbal expression, and then after Marie had another stroke, we worked some more on swallowing. Unfortunately, Marie and I saw each other professionally quite often throughout the '80s. She went in and out of hospitals and grew ever more impaired. Marie's husband, a man in his early nineties, had passed away during the time I treated her. She managed to stay and care for herself in that big, gorgeous home. I'd appointed myself "jack of all trades" in addition to being her therapist and fixed whatever needed repair, moved whatever needed moving, and washed whatever needed washing. We had many laughs together; Marie was a very cool lady.

Despite the fact that Hollywood boasted over 100,000 inhabitants, it was always a small world. I treated my closed head-injury patient, Ken, an active police officer, in his home. I was well along in my second pregnancy. Ken's wife, Sally, was sensitive to my comforts: "Is it too hot in here?" "Does the smell of the bacon bother you?" Sally was an

OB-GY nurse, and it was her face I had woken up to see after my c-section.

An unfriendly rivalry between Jennifer and me for control of our homeowners' association became very awkward when I was sent to treat Jennifer's husband Russ in their home. I had a solid professional reputation and she knew enough not to ask for anyone else to treat a member of her family. Tactfully, Jennifer made it her business to be away from home when I visited—her husband and I worked alone. I knew that Jennifer and Russ's son, a youngish Fort Lauderdale policeman, still lived at home but I never ran into him either. My patient, Russ, had some facial paralysis on one side that I had hoped to lessen with thermo-stimulation and exercises. I went to their freezer to put together a makeshift ice bag. Instead of food, their freezer was filled with dead frozen parakeets. Each little colorful body was individually wrapped in a baggie. Then the birds were stacked neatly into five tiers—a lot of bird bodies. My patient told me they belonged to his son. I thought it was a little creepy.

Strange, too, was the hobby of my millionaire retiree who once owned Miami's famous Jockey Club. There were animal traps behind his mansion on Golden Beach, a very glitzy oceanfront village north of Miami Beach. South Florida property owners with fruit trees in their yards, regardless of the opulence of the neighborhood, are no strangers to big brown rats that fall and drown in pools or sun themselves on peoples' patios. But this millionaire caught and prepared opossums for himself to eat. Yum. A bit chewy and greasy, but it tastes like chicken.

"Bad strange" was seeing purple bumps on my middle-aged gay patient's hands, not knowing in the early eighties that I was treating my first AIDS patient. Creepier to me even than pastel-colored bird bodies: kind of scary, as well, since I had several blood transfusions to prepare me for surgery after my ectopic pregnancy in 1982, fifteen months before my son Ian was born. I nervously kept up with the recommended blood tests for the HIV virus for over a year.

Marilyn was a jovial, earthy woman in her forties when she was felled by a brainstem stroke. The clot rendered her speech muffled, imprecise and nasal. Her palate drooped, totally occluding her pharynx. She was unable to form or effectively move a bolus of food or liquid with her weakened tongue. She was at high risk for aspiration pneumonia with a disrupted inefficient swallow. Marilyn was a woman who loved her food. If I was not going to ease her into safely eating again, she was determined to eat and drink anyway she could. At that time, I didn't have the benefit of technology for diagnosis of the character and extent of a patient's swallowing problem. I did what was then and now called a Bedside Swallow Evaluation. I was treating the way I flew – by dead reckoning. Very gradually, Marilyn resumed eating a modified diet. I recall the easiest foods she could control were canned, overcooked, very soft saucy pastas. When she felt comfortable with the pasta, we moved on to mashed, overcooked vegetables. Then we tried ground meat: ground turkey was easier to manage than the grittier hamburger meat. Marilyn's doctors told her she would not ever be able to regain her ability to swallow. They insisted she get a feeding tube inserted. A feeding tube was not on Marilyn's agenda. Together, we proved her doctors wrong. She remained healthy, got healthier still. She dodged the aspiration bullet.

Two years after my treatment of Marilyn's speech and swallowing, I was invited to her daughter's thirteenth birthday party. Marilyn held court with her and her daughter's closest friends. Her speech was clearer but still had that muffled in-the-head quality. Marilyn was never self-conscious about the way she sounded. She had other priorities. She made a feast of tasty dishes and gorged herself like the rest of her guests.

My Higher Power

Home wasn't a good place for me in the mid-1980s. I looked for help from psychotherapists and attended Al-Anon in a neighborhood church hall. My particular Al-Anon meeting turned out to be a disappointment—the dry drunks sat in one room venting and the family members sat in another room, venting. Our first-name-only circle could have used more ventilation since the put-upon circle of enablers turned to cigarettes much the way the anonymous dry-drunks used alcohol. We sat in a permanent cloud of secondhand fumes.

I rebelled against carrying the label of "alcoholic loved-one." I didn't believe I was an enabler or rescuer or whatever AA called us. I didn't smoke and couldn't breathe in that meeting room. And I did not invest in putting my troubles into a basket called higher power. I was more practical than spiritual. I wanted to know what I should be doing and get on with my life. I had unfinished business with my father's drinking that I felt was ham-stringing me somehow in achieving peace with myself. I had heard about ACOA: Adult Children of Alcoholics and attended a group. My group did not light up. I could breathe. At least until the individuals began to speak, and then I held my breath. But not because of smoke but because of emotion—recognition, relief, memories. My eyes teared up and midway through a gentleman's testimony, as his verbal contribution was called, I lost it and sat sobbing: I was in the right place.

I wiped my eyes with tissue, gained some modicum of control, and stole furtive glances at my fellow ACOAs. We were a well-dressed, turned-out group. No one evinced such total lack of self-esteem that they were slovenly or smelly. This seemed like a much healthier bunch of people than those in my Al-Anon group. Most importantly, the solution seemed to be self-determined. No higher power—I alone was responsible. The well-dressed man I had heard that day talked about his alcoholic father who had disciplined him by trying to drown him in the toilet. That boy grew up to be an over-achiever, hell-bent on proving his worth, becoming a success in life, and yet he always believed he belonged in that toilet. I easily could relate. I attended more groups and bought some books with the ACOA focus on wellness. I began to understand that the damage self-destructive parents may do had to be dealt with, and dealt with constantly, every day, every time that five-year-old's emotions surface and compete with an adult's cognitive self. I needed to take care of me. I needed to forgive me. I needed to love me.

Turning the Page

The nineties was a busy decade. I was a full-time therapist, a full-time student finishing my MBA, and a full-time fiancé planning my second wedding, which would be held in October of 1990.

Home Health was assigning me more and more Hispanic clients.

Miami Dade's hospital patients were mostly Spanish speaking and freshly sick. I made do with what little Spanish I knew treating my swallowing-impaired caseload. But I was floundering trying to treat the subtleties of communication in a language not my own. I gradually moved my assignments farther and farther north, into the northern reaches of Broward County, close to wealthy and privileged Boca Raton and Palm Beach. I took a job in the Hospital District as Coordinator of Speech-Language Services. I taught speech-language pathologists how to perform videofluoroscopic swallow studies. I taught myself the very definite differences between the adult swallowing anatomy and physiology and that of the child. I studied videos of infant swallowing disorders and painstakingly learned how to distinguish a child's anatomical landmarks. I figured out the dynamics of eating in the pediatric population. A co-worker suggested I "switch-hit" and take children into my caseload: she said I would ensure myself of a job in a tight market (for non-Spanish speaking therapists).

My work was dedicated to one hospital. I had a waiting list of pediatric out-patients scheduled and was obligated to treat the pediatric and adult in-patients. I liked doing my swallow studies; I didn't so much like trying to fix autism in children. I grew attached to my cerebral palsy patients and their appreciative parents. I was impatient with the entitled attitude of newly-wealthy twenty-something parents. These youngsters who had profited from the dot-com bubble, became instantly obscenely rich and felt entitled. They brought me their designer-dressed lisping offspring. If they were kept waiting because an earlier session went longer or if I was called upstairs to treat, they bitched. I hated cramming one outpatient child and parent after another while keeping up with very sick inpatients. The job was very stressful.

I learned much in this period so it wasn't a total bust; I learned how to put children, and adults as well, into extension or flexion pattern postures to improve swallowing. I learned how common reflux is in an infant and how to treat an inability to suckle. I learned passive techniques that are useful when children are too ill to perform oral movements. I learned that I could be effective at treating kids even if I preferred to work with adults.

One high point was Dakota, a three-year-old beauty brought to the outpatient clinic by her grandmother. She had the worst case of verbal apraxia* I had seen since I treated my thirty-year-old patient, Ashley, years earlier. Apraxia is a condition—either acquired by stroke, injury or congenital cause—whereby the person does not have the ability to perform an intention. The signal from the "I wish I could…" area of the brain fails to connect with the muscles that make it happen. I was taught that "apraxia of speech" corresponded to an impairment of the production of phonemic sequences, or a series of sounds that make up words, and along with Broca's aphasia was generically called "nonfluent, expressive aphasia."

"The validity of the term apraxia of speech is discussed. The major objection to the term is the implication that the observed phonological impairment is a motor impairment, separate and distinct from other language systems. The rationale for the term is examined from three vantage points: the definitions of the terms aphasia and apraxia of speech, the separation of the phonological symptom complex from other systems necessary for language behavior, and the interpretations of the symptoms themselves. The author concludes that the given definitions of aphasia and apraxia are not that clearly differentiated; that tasks used to demonstrate the adequacy of perceptual acuity were inadequate and did not truly test the required perceptual processes; that the evident influence of other linguistic variables on phonological production demonstrates that there is not a discrete separation of motor activity from other language processes, or their possible impairment (aphasia); and finally, that the various symptoms, taken separately or together, may have alternate interpretations that do not lend themselves to the concept of motor impairment."

Journal of Speech and Hearing Disorders
Vol.39: 53-64 February, 1974.

American Speech-Language-Hearing Association
"Some Objections to the Term Apraxia of Speech"©
~ A. Damien Martin

Three-year old Dakota, who suffered from this condition, was functionally mute. She didn't utter a sound. I channeled Ashley and used blowing, spitting, noisemakers, blow-toys, party favors, horns—anything in my imagination to jump-start her voice. When I got sound, I went to consonants, one-by-tedious-one. I gave her a bowl of dried peas. I asked her to move them pea-by-pea from that bowl into another. Every time she picked up a pea, she had to say, "puh!" then "pea" then "peapod," etc. When she entered pre-school later that year, she had a respectable arsenal of words at her disposal, enough for sure for her new SLP to build upon.

Another two-year-old client of mine, sweet little Rambo (really!), started speaking with a substantial stutter. His mother brought him to my outpatient clinic. I quickly read all the material I could find on childhood stuttering. I was hardly the seasoned stuttering expert. In fact, my only stutterer was the unfortunate man I had met while a graduate student, and he knew more than I did. I discovered that this little guy fancied himself quite the rock star, so I asked his mother to let Rambo bring in his guitar to the next session. That guitar was bigger than he was.

Rambo dragged that guitar in, sat down in his little plastic chair, and strummed some notes. As he strummed, I made up silly nonsense phrases that I put to tune. He played and I chanted away, "I love your guitar! I want a hamburger with ketchup! Where is your little brother?" I encouraged him to use lots and lots of air to sing. Pretty soon he began to make up silly stuff too. He never stuttered while he strummed his guitar. I called this to his attention, that his talking was smooth when he was with the guitar. I asked him to try to make without-guitar-talking just as smooth. He could.

Skip and I decided to sell the house I had bought with my first husband eighteen years before to move to a less-congested neighborhood and a roomier home in Plantation Acres, Florida. My Hollywood Hills house sheltered me during SWAT teams scouting hostage neighbors. My near-death ruptured ectopic pregnancy and later the birth of my precious son Ian. The terrible sickness and death of my mother. Through the years spent building a successful private practice. Meeting, then marrying, my true love, Skip. Nothing prepared me for the adventure of selling my house.

My realtor scheduled an open house for potential buyers to scope out the place. The front door was left open to welcome in prospective buyers. I had also left one of the patio doors open so my beautiful blooming orchids could be seen. My realtor was greeting newcomers in the living room. I turned away from them, trying to look nonchalant and caught a glimpse of a rapidly moving object on the floor. A fruit rat had run into the house from the open patio door. I *was not* in the habit of having vermin in my house! In his panic, the rat turned the corner and ran in the bedroom area *at the same time* that the realtor and the couple crossed into the kitchen. What happened next was a blend of *I Love Lucy* and *The Keystone Cops.* I ran looking for the rat and the rat ran out a door into the kitchen a heartbeat behind the couple turning into the bedroom hallway. This comedy routine went on forever, it seemed. The couple never saw the rat, we scared the rat out of the house, and eventually sold our house—ratless—to a nice, single lady.

Tighter, stricter Medicare regulations were making earning a living in home health unattractive. Too much paperwork, evaluate then see the patient for a week or two at the most, less work for speech-language pathologists as the government apparently thought we were unnecessary. I decided to cut my losses in my private practice, quit my separate contracts and take a job in a nursing home that functioned as a 'transitional care facility.' I went from lab-coat-skirt-and-blouse to scrubs. I didn't mind going to work in pajamas.

Traditional nursing homes were caring places where folks brought loved ones they themselves could not care for. These loved ones had conditions that required 24/7 nursing care. The bill for this nursing care was absorbed by Medicare, in some states Medicaid or families paid privately. When Medicare/Medicaid laws changed, nursing home beds were held for private payers. This forced many people to care for their sick loved ones at home since the cost could be prohibitive. Home health made that more possible.

As nursing homes emptied, they needed to retool to accept the people who were discharged from the hospital but continued to need "skilled nursing care." Soon, "skilled nursing care" incorporated "skilled rehabilitation." Wings of many nursing homes were dedicated to "transitional care"—a transition between the hospital and home. The residents of the nursing home were typically in a separate wing. A patient soon-to-leave his/her hospital room would be given the options of getting a full day of intensive therapy or a minimal of three hours of therapy. Free-standing or hospital-owned rehabilitation centers would provide intensive all day PT/OT/ST. The nursing homes accepted those patients who could only perform about three hours of therapy.

I reported to a lovely lady named Cassondra who was twenty-five—twenty years younger than me. She was lovely during the initial interview, as I am sure I was, and then she later let her fangs show. She was also a speech pathologist who didn't treat patients, but led a rehab department. I truly don't know if Cassondra resented that I had more experience than she did. Or perhaps she was exercising control over an older employee. Or maybe she was just bat-poop crazy. Dunno. She second-guessed my diagnoses and treatments. She questioned my methods. She overturned the decisions I'd made. She asserted that her own opinion prevail over mine in how to manage the caseload she assigned me. She then began criticizing me publicly. *What is it with younger SLP's in supervisory positions?* I wondered.

Fortunately, the rehab placement company that supplied therapists (and me) to this nursing home, invited me to apply as the supervisor of speech services in several high end nursing establishments in three Florida counties. I left Cassondra's nursing home and happily left Cassondra behind. I was back in dresses, heels, and a lab coat. I liked the travel, the time I spent listening to music in my car as I drove between facilities. I liked my co-supervisors of physical and occupational therapies. I liked mentoring young therapists. I did not like the bureaucracy of a corporation. I hated the paperwork and petty rules. I didn't like reporting to younger managers. I thought my bosses were mean and stupid. I was more than ever authority-challenged. I missed my own business.

Hadn't I learned anything? Some months later, the company went belly-up and I was on my own once more.

The mid-1990s were a blur in my career. I no longer had my dependable private practice and its diligently collected contracts to sustain me. I took one full-time position after another and none of them was satisfying. I balked at trying to fit into a corporate mold. Friends told me again and again that I had made a huge mistake: that working for oneself for twenty years makes one a lousy employee. But then there was the work and my patients.

I explored getting out of the Speech Pathology field. I loved aviation, so maybe I could get yet another degree and design airports. But I decided that it required too much school. I thought I could be a flight attendant, but then decided that forty-seven was too old to start. Maybe I'd become a day trader on the stock exchange and make a lot of money. But I tried that and failed expensively. I took whatever contract jobs various placement people offered me, working in outpatient rehab centers and group homes.

So while my work life stagnated, I ended up trying something totally outside my parameters. In the fall of 2000, I adopted a potbellied pig.

Pigs had fascinated me ever since I had been a child observing my uncle's few farm animals. My mother's brother had come to live with us from the Ukraine. He kept a handful of rabbits, a goat and two pigs in pens he built in our side-yard. I was about eight or nine, always a feral kind of kid who wandered for hours alone in the forests. But I loved following Uncle Andrew around, learning what mushrooms to pick and how to care for the animals.

One of his two pigs was always breaking out of the pen and he couldn't understand how. No holes were dug, no fence was broken, no door opened. I hid and watched the pigs at play in their pen. In time, one sidled up to the fence and rubbed its body on it, much like my uncle did when he had an itch and couldn't reach it with his hand. Then the pig stood there a moment, stock-still. His buddy strolled over, climbed onto his back and jumped over the four-foot fence. Pigs used strategy. I was fascinated. I didn't know much more about pigs, but the pig I would come to raise would become the teacher I needed to help me learn the reality of my future, profoundly affected patients—the Sumter residents.

Through the years, I had collected piggy banks, stuffed piggy toys, pig noses that were worn over one's own, pig calendars, etc. At county fairs, the animals I was most attracted to were the pigs. I even liked the movie, *Babe*. I am not alone in my appreciation of the pig— George Orwell and Charlotte (of Web fame), as well as many potbellied pig owners share the same appreciation.

Fast forward to 2000. A physical therapist friend of mine who had a ranch out on the Western borders of the Everglades came to visit me one day. She hoisted a box out of her car and brought it over.

"The owner of a petting zoo lives next door to me. Her pig just had another litter and they don't have room for more pigs. Are you interested in adopting one of these four?"

"Certainly not!" I told her. While I loved pigs, I had two dogs and several cats at last count, and I didn't want another mouth to feed. Stuffed or plastic pigs were one thing, a live pig was another.

"Could you just keep one or two overnight? They're only two weeks old and they stay in the box. Please give just one a home for the night and I'll find a permanent home for these little cuties tomorrow. Just keep one overnight."

I agreed to take just one little piggy. For just one night. And little piggy stayed.

Her name became Pegasus or "Peggy" for short. A mere two weeks old, she fit in the crook of my arm. She was black all over except for her big pink nose and a white blaze down the middle of her face. A Latino friend declared that the white blaze on Peg's head was a symbol of good luck. Peggy did little else besides drink, pee, sleep—and scream!!—the first week or two. Baby pig's screams are intensely ear-shattering.

I questioned our good luck.

We were promised that Peggy, "certified" by the owners of the petting zoo was a "teacup" Vietnamese potbellied pig, and would only grow to thirty-five pounds. My experience with pigs from my childhood made me very skeptical. Livestock boars and sows grew larger than seven-hundred pounds. Come what may, my family and I were smitten with this little Pegasus pig and we promised that we would continue to love and care for her even if she grew enormous. "I'll still love you when you're old and fat," we promised each other.

Initially, we could not give her the run of the fenced in dog pen just outside the garage; she was way too tiny to be entrusted with the curious and territorial dogs. She lived for a month in a dog crate filled with pieces of rags for her to nest in. The crate had a door so Miss Peg could be contained. We kept the crate in my home office at first then moved it downstairs to our formal dining room that was seldom used. We chaperoned her visits in the dog pen and were charmed when our big Dalmatian drank side-by-side with little missy Peg. Our Labrador Retriever, Havoc, was the nurturer—he took it upon himself to make sure Peggy stayed close, didn't wander, and didn't explore his dog toys. After she played a while with the dogs and did her bathroom business, Peg was returned to the metal dog crate in our for-the-most-part-unused formal dining room.

Two-week-old Peg became housebroken very easily. We researched that miniature pigs like to use cedar chips instead of stuff like cat litter. We got a small "litter-pan," a large plastic tray with high sides, and filled it with cedar chips. After a moment or two of sniffing, Peg peed in the pee-pan. It was amazing since the dogs still had accidents in the house during their adult years. Peg was fed out of a flat plastic bowl. She started on formula much the same as a human baby feeds on formula in infancy. She then progressed to piglet mash (found at feed stores). She had a habit of sniffing her food and then overturning the bowl and licking the food from the mess on the floor. But we were not going to let her do that in our dining room. My husband, Skip, got an eighteen-inch by two-foot plywood board and hammered down a three-by-six board onto one end, forming a right angle. We bought a water bowl that was designed to attach with a plastic screw onto a parrot's cage. The idea was that Peg would stand on the flat board and eat from the bowl which was secured to the right angle board.

Peggy watched from the other side of her dining room while Skip put the bowl on the long board and stuck the protruding end through a round hole he made in the standing up board. He then reinforced the bowl onto the board by screwing it on with the plastic bolt. We had finally made a mess-proof way of feeding Peg in the house—a bowl that she could not overturn. Peggy waited until this contraption was finished, ambled over to it and giving Skip what looked like a wink, used her nose to turn the screwed bolt, removed the bowl and flipped it. Pigs have brains.

Pigs have habits that are very different from dogs or cats, and my family was determined to learn "pig." Initially, Peg did not like to be handled. She screamed louder than a 747. Since we had her in the midst of our living space, we needed to reinforce play time, sleep time and quiet time. Forcing ourselves on Peg didn't cut it: she broke our eardrums. We needed to woo her. We needed to learn to speak pig.

Raising a tiny, baby potbellied pig was novel and very rewarding. But Peggy Pig didn't pay all the bills, although in time she contributed. My husband and I were in agreement that we had to leave Florida. His work was affected by his inability to speak Spanish, as mine was. We waited until Ian graduated high school then put our house up for sale. When Ian left for university that fall, we moved out as well.

PART THREE

NORTH TO SOUTH CAROLINA

Transitions

After twenty-six years in Broward County, it was time to leave. One thing after another had kept me in the area during that time—my mother, my first marriage, and my son. Then after my divorce from my son's father, I wanted to stay close so that my son could grow up with both of his parents nearby. The two-parent couples (me and my new spouse, my ex and his) attended my son's high school graduation, and then Skip and I immediately put the For Sale sign on the front lawn. I loved my house, my neighborhood, and my lifestyle, but without work there would be no house and no lifestyle. I'd have to find a new neighborhood.

We had considered several places to relocate—some cities in California, some cities in Colorado close to dear friends, but in the end, we decided to stay on the East Coast. Most of Skip's family lived on the East Coast, and I had family and close friends nearby.

We had been vacationing in the spring of 2000. It was a way to get away, but also to explore possible relocation sites. We had planned to stay in a bed-and-breakfast in Davidson, north of Charlotte, North Carolina. We had been there before and found it attractive. The plan then was to proceed into the mountains of North Carolina to Blowing Rock, also a place we were familiar with from past vacations. Blowing Rock and nearby Boone were possible contenders for home. We flew to Atlanta and rented a car. We drove up I-85 to Charlotte. Between Atlanta and Charlotte was the upstate of South Carolina. Living in New York and visiting Florida entailed driving down and back through the east coast of South Carolina. My impression of South Carolina (through most of my twenties) was that it was a South of the Border (the name of an actual place), tacky, faux-Mexican collection of service stations, souvenir shops, and a snack bar. Then, a boring landscape of Stuckey's locations and firecracker stores. I hadn't put South Carolina on any short or long list of places to consider moving to.

Two hours out of Atlanta, we crossed the border into the upstate of South Carolina. It was surprisingly hilly with views of the Smokey Mountains to the north. When we got hungry, we looked for an exit off of I-85 that might host a restaurant or two. Just past a sign for Clemson, South Carolina were a number of exits advertising a place named Greenville. We figured with multiple exits, we could find a decent place to lunch.

Every state, it seems, has its Greenville. But Greenville, South Carolina had a beautiful downtown off one of those exits. It was midday on a Tuesday and people dressed in business attire were lunching at sidewalk cafes. After we ate, we strolled downtown and admired much of what this town offered—a tree-lined Main Street with plenty of inexpensive as well as upscale eateries, jewelry stores, clothing stores, offices, and apartments—which kept people in the downtown area after business hours. Greenville was...perfect.

When we got home we Googled Greenville, wrote to the Chamber of Commerce, and researched the town thoroughly. One or both of us went back and stayed several days to see if it was real or a mirage. We were warned by friends that Greenville was the buckle of the Bible belt—very Republican, very Southern, and perhaps inhospitable to Yankees. But the upstate of South Carolina was also becoming very international with BMW and Michelin bringing in workers. We took a chance.

I applied for and got a job in South Carolina immediately, before leaving Florida. I flew in for the interview in an office building in downtown Greenville. I had another day for house-hunting. My realtor gave me a stack of prospective homes for sale. I "curbed" neighborhoods with my list of "For Sales" in hand and found a great piece of property. I made an offer without even showing the house to my husband. I just told him, "Relax, Dear, there are five garages."

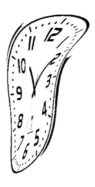

Sumter Center 2002

The want ad on the Internet said something like, "Certified Speech-Language Pathologist wanted for full-time position with adults. Experience with swallowing and neurological deficits required." I don't recall what else it said but it most certainly did not mention drool.

My first day of work. I took the Interstate a ways. I exited and passed miles of woodlands punctuated by a couple of rusted single-wide trailers and some deer stands. My directions took me to a road with a long pink wall, upon which a sign said "Sumter Center." That wall seemed to go on for a bit, maybe a good half-mile or so.

A paved driveway in and a guardhouse interrupted the wall; one could not see further than that. I could see no explanation; I supposed it was a rehabilitation hospital, like the one in which I worked in Westchester County. I was hesitant about going in right away, so I drove around the property to explore. At an intersection with another two-lane blacktop, the pink wall stopped and was replaced by a tall wrought-iron fence that stretched along that road for another half-mile or so. Inside here I could see paved streets, some trees, a fenced in swimming pool, and a collection of plain, rectangular buildings in a row. Oddly, I didn't see any people.

Sumter Center had opened in 1966, one of a chain of mental health facilities throughout the Southeast. The Sumter Centers were involved in the treatment of the mentally and physically impaired, and specialized in children. Their mission was to provide treatment services for essentially development delays, and to support these individuals in the attainment of "desired personal outcomes." Sumter housed these individuals in thirty-six cottages on 168.5 acres near Spartanburg, South Carolina.

I am not likely to forget the first day of work at Sumter. I turned into that paved driveway, presented my name at the guardhouse, and followed the road along the wrought-iron fence I had explored on the other side. I still didn't know the purpose of this place. Only that it was a community for impaired adults. I was a bit apprehensive not knowing what I was about to sign up for.

I found the speech building easily—my new boss, Ellen, gave good directions. It was one of the plain rectangular buildings that I peeked at through the wrought iron fence. Close up, I was dismayed at the condition of the building—and the entire campus. The place looked old and unkempt. The entrances to each building were gated and chain-locked with seriously thick iron chains. Ellen, a speech-language pathologist, met me at the speech office and asked if I wanted a tour. She had a distinct twinkle in her eye and said, "Let's see if you stay."

We got into her car—I would've walked, but she said it was too far. We were off to see the campus. Because this place was a community populated by adults over the age of twenty-one who lived on the campus permanently, they were "residents" not "patients." The population of Sumter was labeled 'multiply handicapped.' They lived in charming pastel-colored single cottages with front and back porches accessed by two or three steps, or a ramp. Each was set at intervals along short streets off two, long boulevards. In addition to the resident cottages, the community contained a permanent fire substation, a large gym complete with basketball court, and a bowling alley along with the various out-buildings used for therapy or administration, and a large hangar-looking workshop employing many of the residents. Although the community once held a small working farm, this was gone by the time I started working there. The residents and staff never lost their love for whatever animals wandered—or were brought—in.

I saw no one around. The campus was completely deserted. We turned a corner and I saw fleeting movement in the corner of my eye. When I turned to look, I saw someone crawl out of an oversized garbage bag, spilling the contents along with him. He went back and grabbed for something and stood up, eating his find. Appalled, I said "Ellen! We have to stop him, he's eating garbage!" She just smiled. I think of that first impression because over time I had come to be pretty used to people eating litter, feces, stuffed animals, clothing, underwear, sponges, other people, and themselves. It was a gradual thing, daily shocks that inured one to just about anything. I discovered that these people had a different set of boundaries than I did. Rather than being disgusted, I was fascinated. I set out to try and figure out these folks and their boundaries.

The basic criterion for admission to Sumter Center was the label "mentally retarded." In time, this was changed to "mentally challenged," and then to a more acceptable but very misleading term, "developmentally delayed." As if in time they would catch up. They were 'delayed.' When they turn, say, fifty, they will catch up and they'll be just the same as you and me. The reality is that when brains are broken, folks cannot learn abstractions, or solve the most basic of problems, and they have poor coping skills in a faster paced "average" world. The friends I made at Sumter Center were also autistic-like, schizophrenic-like, behaviorally challenged, inappropriate, weird. I say "like" because essentially their performance skills were not testable. Their performances could only be observed and rated.

They presented characteristics of those who are formally labeled "autistic" or "schizophrenic" in addition to "all of the above," a veritable hodge-podge of Axis I and II labels. The Diagnostic and Statistical Manual of Mental Disorders divides psychiatric manifestations into five groups. The first two describe the disorders. Axis I includes clinical syndromes, or, essentially, "the diagnosis." Some of the Axis I clinical syndromes include depression, schizophrenia, bipolar disorder. Axis II disorders are underlying: pervasive or personality disorders such as Schizoid Personality Disorder, Paranoid Personality Disorder, Borderline Personality Disorder and mild mental retardation. Autism spectrum disorders used to be categorized as Axis II but were reclassified in Axis I. Some psychiatrists put severe mental retardation into Axis I as a developmental disorder, or a disorder first diagnosed in infancy or childhood. I don't understand why mental retardation is split into severe and mild with one form in Axis I and the other in Axis II.

Sometimes a person has no Axis I or II diagnosis, but falls into Axis III. Axis III includes physical conditions or non-psychiatric disorders which impact the Axis I and II disorders. These would be brain injury or HIV/AIDS, for instance. Axis IV describes the events that impact Axis I and II, and the severity of psychosocial forces on the ability to function. Axis V describes the person's highest level of functioning, scored on a scale of 0-100 on a Global Assessment of Functioning and Children's Global Assessment (<18 years).

Members of the staff at Sumter would bicker with each other as to what to label a resident—autistic, pica (a strong desire to eat nonfood items), delayed, hallucinatory. It was all intellectual masturbation. It did not matter for the State of South Carolina's funding and placement purposes. Legally, Sumter residents were diagnosed as having an Axis I, Mental Retardation diagnosis. Behaviorally, some demonstrated autism or schizophrenia. Some of the formal psychiatric diagnoses included in the Diagnostic and Statistical Manual of Mental Disorders were also mutually exclusive of another. For instance, one cannot be both "bipolar" and have a "major depression disorder" because major depression was part of the diagnosis of bipolar.

Another example based on duration or severity is schizophrenia versus schizophreniform disorder. Regardless of the medical formalities, regardless of the characteristic of the disorder, regardless of the hours of bickering among the community's professionals as to the residents' behavior, the bottom line was that each of these folks was "broken." For the majority, their brain damage was congenital: it was a result of genes or of birth. They couldn't be compared with infants, children or animals. Some could be taught rudimentary skills, others could not. Some carried heavy psychological baggage, and would strike out physically and randomly. Being in the same room with a violent, defiant, fearful and agitated resident was obviously necessary to teaching or treating him. Add 'adult, bulky, strong' to violent and irrational and personal contact became risky and dangerous. Injury to staff was a daily, nay, hourly occurrence—it went with the territory. You learned to dodge or "gently restrain."

I want to explain why I consider some of the individuals I met at Sumter "friends." In order to do this, I have to recount for you my journey of enlightenment. Please understand that much of what I say here is *mine*. I don't pretend to be socially acceptable, politically correct, or tactful. I call 'em as I see 'em and I believe that in this way I have come to an understanding, in fact a great appreciation for and respect of some of the residents I have served.

How could I write about Sumter? Each day I recall brings me a new image, a new realization. I could start with the multisensory room. Many of the more behaviorally challenged residents were regularly brought to the multisensory room to calm down and relax. The therapists used the multisensory room for Sensory Integration treatment. Different seating opportunities, lights and music, a ball pit, darkness or swings were available to shape a person's behavior in order to rudimentarily socialize or teach. Patients could relax and chill here. The therapists could use some activity the resident liked as reinforcement for a job well done.

The sign outside the multisensory room reads Take Off Your Shoes. I opened the door slowly, not knowing what to expect. The room was dark. I felt as disoriented as I did when I would enter a movie theatre to look for seats after the lights have gone off.

Then, a light here, some color there. Darks forms morph into bodies and into the most fantastic shapes: humans contorted into positions that are unimaginable even to my younger self doing back bends or somersaults. A revolving light passes, illuminating a monster.

What did this person's mother think when he was born? Did she stay to see him grow up into a boy not much taller than an infant? I wondered.

An infant with tiny feet and stiff arms jutting out at the sides like a broken kite jammed into the box it came in. A man/boy with a face so disturbing I couldn't help but stare. A grown man now who screams endlessly and randomly.

"Hi Rick!"

I greet him when I recognize him. Eyes shaded by thick brows look up, search, and finally find my face—well at least one of the eyes does, the other perhaps preoccupied with inner thoughts.

Rick laid on a slanted, padded board, feet akimbo on either side of a padded, large triangular-shaped mat, with arms that flailed at his sides, his neck bounced unsupported on the uppermost of the slant. The pads glistened with fresh drool. A psychedelic flashing strobe turned his body yellow first, and then magenta. I realized he didn't look any less weird in magenta. I stepped back and hit my heel on another human.

This one was a female form, lying in a fetal position, rocking. Her head looked like it had been attacked by mange. Hair squirted in clumps, interrupted by fresh scabs. The face shocked because it was…just a face, rather ordinary, maybe pretty at times. She wore a different shoe on each of her feet. Thankfully, I noted that there were only two feet—there were no freaks here with limbs duplicated or missing, just run-of-the-mill freaks who scared kids on the outside.

A man sat cross-legged on a large air mattress and bounced in time to the music piped into the room. This was rare—he was not always quiet; in his cottage he rarely sat still. Next to him there was a man whom I somehow recognized—he looked like an uncle, maybe, or someone's neighbor. He was wearing a karate helmet so he didn't do permanent damage when he threw himself head first onto the ground, which he did in ritualized intervals. In between there was a series of seemingly random moves: he smacked his face, turned his head sharply, pulled on his pants, rubbed the middle finger of his left hand on his groin, and then licked his finger. He dove onto the floor, smacked, sharply turned, pulled his pants, rubbed his groin, licked his finger, dove. And then continued in the same fashion.

The woman across the room was searching the floor on her hands and knees. She pounced and put whatever she found in her mouth. Investigation revealed a staple, which she would not release. She swallowed it and repeated the search on the floor. It was rumored that she once ate her own bra. I wonder if she chewed a little at a time or all at once. *How do you imagine the unimaginable?* I asked myself.

In the corner was a figure of undetermined gender lit by a waterfall of delicate glass lights which turned pink and then blue, then green, and then pink once more. It was motionless, but keened softly and hypnotically.

A short man wandered into the darkness with a magazine rolled in his hand. He visited each of the other forms, one who kicked at him to leave, and another who reached out and pulled at his clothes. He asked by gesture for something to write with, despite that he cannot write. His ears were cauliflowered—but actually there were really no ears on his head, just lumpy flesh without holes. He was bald with scabs and sores on his dome, a dome which ellipsed at the forehead so much that he had a shelf over his eyes, a shelf of forehead. He had one eye but when he smiled his silly little face lit up, making anyone seeing him smile, too. I was told he was only a boy during hurricane Hugo and lived with his parents near Charleston. Their house blew off and the parents, desperate to save their son from injury or certain death, tied him to a tree. He was found still tied to his tree days after the hurricane departed, which left little else besides that tree and the boy, still standing. The boy, then almost nine, never said another word. He lost his eye, too, had periods of blank stares, and asked for water constantly by pointing to his mouth.

I *loved* working at Sumter. I enjoyed my fellow therapists, and have held many close then, and long after I left. The many levels of workers at the community naturally spoke English—a huge advantage because it was difficult to rehabilitate someone's language when you don't speak or understand it. I also loved the challenge of totally changing my career path and learning new skills with an amazingly novel population. And I loved Ellen. She was the first supervisor who showed me respect, encouragement and friendship—and she, too, was a speech-language pathologist. My record of working under other SLPs had been dismal to that point.

Gerry and Sean

Eunice, my occupational therapist friend, and I were returning to her car from a meeting in the administration area of the campus. From a distance I saw a resident physically abusing a staff member.

I was almost about to say something when Eunice yelled, "Oh my god! It's Gerry!"

"Who?" I said. "It's Gerry!" she repeated.

I concentrated, trying to see what the hell was happening. Gerry was very agitated and the staff member didn't know how to handle him. Gerry was a well-muscled 5'8" man who was known to "go off" at any moment and become violent.

Since I seemed to be one of few who could calm Gerry down, Eunice said, "I'll let you out here—go help him. He will listen to you."

I got out, walked over to Gerry, and stood still. Then, I quietly extended my hand out to him. Gerry calmed right down and took my hand. I felt, well, justifiably great to be able to relate to this severely autistic man. I had spent months and months figuring out Gerry's reinforcers and preferences in the sensory integration room. I allowed him time to sniff doorways and lick walls and drop down to the ground to press his groin into the ground, as this was his regular routine as he walked through the campus. I waited out his rituals. It was part of my respect for him.

He came back to take my hand each time. He walked very docilely. I was impressed; Eunice and I had done a great job of Sensory Integration. When we got to his workroom, there was some sort of commotion.

Someone said, "Don't go in!" but Gerry already had the door open and was entering. It was then that I saw the piles of human poop in a line to the door. Gerry did not hesitate—he dropped to his stomach and put his tongue into the closest pile. I started screaming, repulsed. What the hell was my frame of reference for feces eating? My mother taught me to wipe front to back, after all. Well, so much for S.I. and bollocks to my knowledge of my residents.

I accumulated many cookies on the Internet in my quest to understand why people would be drawn to consuming their own feces. Individuals who collect covert information on the Internet on the general public for the purposes of spying or marketing or what-have-you, would have a ball classifying me on the basis of my searches. Google "coprophilia" and you get led to some interesting porn sites.

Sumter Center was fortunate to have an expensively equipped sensory integration lab/multisensory room. I seriously doubt the staff would have been effective at training the more behaviorally-challenged residents without it.

We can understand sensory integration's rationale: being calm allows us to be alert and alert enables us to attend. Attending helps us learn. We solve our immediate sensory discomfort issues so that we can pay better attention: we grab a sweater, a glass of water, escape to the restroom, jiggle our feet, or pop our knuckles. But autistics have impaired senses, and have a much harder time filtering extra stimuli out of their environments; focusing attention is a major challenge. No attention, no learning. Getting folks to focus is that important. The center of the Sumter universe, therefore, became "the multisensory room" or otherwise named "the S.I. lab." The people involved in using the S.I. Lab to best advantage were first the occupational therapists, then the speech therapists, and finally the cottage caregivers who brought their charges there just to chill out. I, too, used the multisensory room to chill out and sensory integration taught me a great deal about people with all sorts of brains.

∾

143

Sean was a feral child and remained a feral adult. I suppose today he would be described as severely autistic, but feral better describes him. He does not attend to others, but windmills his arms to clear some room around himself. If some hapless individual wanders into his way, they would get smacked and inevitably avoid him. Sean was generally avoided by staff, visitors, and other residents because of this windmilling behavior. Sean did not intend to hurt—he just didn't want others too close. Home staff, who have known him through the years and essentially raised him, would say they don't really know him, that he doesn't seem to listen or relate to them. He would crawl on the floor or spin around in circles, or get around by bending over and backing out of a room. Sean didn't speak.

While his cottage-mates learned to sit at a table on a chair and use utensils (for the most part) to feed themselves, Sean ate his meals from a dish on the floor or where ever he felt like it. Occasionally he joined the others at the table—for a nanosecond. He was diagnosed as a person with severe autism.

Ever loving a good challenge, Eunice and I led Sean into the S.I. room. If we could only fine tune Sean's vestibular system and provide the sensations that he craved, we thought we might be able to go further and establish some sort of interaction with him. At first he wouldn't go in; he was apprehensive, perhaps, about entering the room, so we kept the lights on, despite that the room was designed to be dark with visually captivating individual light designs throughout.

Sean ventured in and stopped at the spinner device on the floor closest to the entrance. This was a solid wood or plastic disk mounted on another disc, which allowed it to hold an adult and rotate by hand. It was spun for him but he appeared unimpressed. Objects were placed on the spinner so its movement was more clearly seen. Sean was curious enough to explore it. He waited for us to move away to another task. He hand-spun the disk once or twice, and then attempted to lie down on it. He was spun clear off the disk and laid there warily. It took several sessions of hand spinning objects, touching and then mounting the disk for him to finally sit on it and allow us to spin him around and around first this way then that. Before long, he learned to spin himself on the spinner.

The room also contained a sturdy "spinner" suspended from the ceiling. The proper name for this apparatus was vestibulator. I guess the name referred to achieving dizziness. It functioned and looked a bit like a swing on a playground except that it moved in all directions, not just back and forward. Sean's feet could not reach the ground—he stayed off the suspended apparatus. But we couldn't keep him off the floor spinner.

Sean spun on and on, but never got dizzy. He bent low. He lay on his back. He craned his neck and leaned to the side. Sean was like Baryshnikov, a veritable ballet-meister on the spinner. He needed to swat us out of the way less and less. To our amazement, he courteously moved the spinner clear of furniture and people, and spun on and on. Maybe it wasn't courtesy, maybe he was tired of getting hung up on something and having to interrupt spinning to free the board. Getting him out of the S.I. room that day took several people because he did not want to leave. He was hooked.

Subsequent visits revealed a Sean more open to exploring his environment. The lights were eventually turned off and Sean tolerated the abrupt change in visibility. He looked at and felt everything in the room. He eventually climbed on the vestibulator and rocked in the puffy rocker. But Sean always returned to his spinner. Seated near to him, Eunice and I chanted "Spin, Sean, Spin!" and were rewarded by an echoing verbal "Spin!" from Sean. To the best of our knowledge "spin" was appropriately Sean's very first word in his thirty-five years. We were euphoric.

Sometime after several weeks, one of us brought potato chips into the S.I. room only to have Sean lunge after them. He learned to ask for chips by imitating the basic functional sign of tapping on his lips. Sean has since repeated the verbal "eat" request, and more than a few times would at least grunt to imitate if not say "eat" clearly. Sean would follow one of us out of his program area or cottage to go to the S.I. Lab if we told him, "Spin Sean!" He docilely would accompany us into the S.I. room, ambulating upright and straight ahead.

I was able to massage his back. No small feat with a person who is repelled by touch. He has provided me with eye contact as he hands me an object that I've requested by holding out my palm. His direct care staff has told me that he is calmer and easier to handle. Coincidence? Perhaps. But what would be next? Could we train Sean with more signs, more words? Why not? His most basic gravitational and vestibular needs were being addressed. He had more opportunity to deal with other things, like asking for food.

Caregivers would commonly help some of the more damaged residents to make peanut butter and jelly sandwiches. The motivation was there: they got food. The lesson was there: first do this and then do that, which taught some residents basic sequencing skills. The facility was there: one had to handle bread, jars, and butter knife appropriately and with an end in sight.

One day, Eunice and I decided that making PB&J sandwiches would be a worthwhile "job" for both Gerry and Sean. Part of the building that housed the speech department also housed a fully-equipped kitchen and large dining area for meetings, a snack area for caregivers, as well as for activities of daily living for those residents showing an aptitude for basic kitchen skills.

Getting both men into the kitchen was challenging enough, sort of like corralling chickens when they don't have any idea where they are being led to and why. Both men just knew they were doing something that was not in their routine, and that made them a bit difficult to handle. Sean thought he should first get acquainted with his environment so he spun around the perimeter of the room touching everything he could with his hands and the bottoms of his feet. Gerry chose an alternative method: he licked the walls and the floor. After this productive period of reconnaissance, both men were led to the table and seated—briefly. Reconnaissance apparently was not yet over.

Seated again for a moment, both men were introduced to white bread, a jar of peanut butter, a jar of jelly, a plate and a butter knife. The act of erecting a peanut butter and jelly sandwich was demonstrated by Eunice, while I narrated. Eunice took Gerry and I tutored Sean. Gerry needed only demonstration and the promise of *food* to create a respectable PB&J sandwich. It took about ten minutes to make and a heartbeat for him to shove it all in his mouth and swallow it whole. Sean didn't quite get the hang of make-a-sandwich. He repeatedly rose to spin around the room, on occasion knocking appliances and plates to the floor. Sean was having none of sitting at a table, taking a lesson or eating. It was Not-in-His-Routine.

Gabriel

Upon starting my work at Sumter Center, I was issued a master key, which I wore on a lanyard around my neck. I was told not to wear it visibly. I tucked it into the neckline of my shirt. The key unlocked the chained gates to the therapy buildings as well as to staff bathrooms, classrooms, workshop rooms, the sensory integration room, and the gym. The reason for the key became obvious—some places needed to be off-limits to some of the residents. Keeping the key beneath my shirt was also made clear the first time a resident grabbed it and pulled me off my feet.

When I arrived for work each day, I entered through the now familiar pink concrete wall down a long drive past the guardhouse, hung a right and drove parallel to the tall, wrought-iron fence past the chapel and the swimming pool to the first therapy building. I stepped over whatever resident was lying in front of the gate, took out my key, and let myself into the outside gate which was secured by a heavy, rusted circle of chain.

Once inside the entry, I used my key again to access the speech department's quarters: generous four rooms of storage, a fridge and microwave, treatment room, communal office, and Ellen's office. Ellen, who was the department manager, had her own large room and two computers. Our speech department offices were generous but not lavish; the building may have been built in the sixties. The floor was concrete and stained. The walls had peeling, no doubt, lead paint. In the summer, we had no shortage of mildew, which grew up the walls in an expanding Rorschach. We shared the building with several rooms that were used as workshops. Some select, more-capable residents worked in these workshops putting packaging together, an example of which is the prepackaged napkin, spork, and salt and pepper available in fast food places.

Around the back of the building, away from the parking area was the gym and the kitchen and dining room for teaching purposes and for the staff. Around the other hallway, more workshop rooms, the bathrooms (mold-covered and stinky from the humidity) and the sensory integration room. Next to our building was another identical building which housed more workshop rooms, communal lounge-type rooms, and the physical and occupational therapy suites.

The individual who usually lay on the ground to block my entry to the speech office was a twenty-something man who looked to be either Middle-Eastern or Hispanic, he went by the name of "Gabe," short for Gabriel. Gabe sat cross-legged much of the time and rocked back and

147

forth with his head down. When someone approached, he looked up to investigate and then quickly down again without any sign of greeting. I was informed he was "severe" and "nonverbal" and always had had a behavior problem.

I always said, "Hi Gabe," whenever I passed him. After several months, I received a short grunt in response. Several more months passed, and Gabe started to rise, follow me into my office, and stand looking at me before flapping his hands before departing to sit cross-legged by the door. I began to engage Gabe in more than just hello. "Would you like a drink of water?" and "How do you feel today?" Ellen reiterated that Gabe did not speak and was likely profoundly disabled.

I inquired of the staff about Gabe at one of our grand round meetings. I was curious about his background and how he ended up at Sumter. The response bowled me over. In the early nineties police came upon a migrant worker, thought to be a fruit picker in the previous decade, sitting beneath a highway overpass. He was holding a woman's dead body. I was told that Gabe's father had thrown his mother off the I-85 overpass. Apparently, he had second thoughts about his feelings for his wife because he continued to hold her. I don't know if that detail is true. Certainly the corpse-clutching man under the overpass is true because the papers reported it, but whether there was a direct connection to an abandoned child placed by the state in Sumter Center is conjecture. Regardless, Gabe had been a recently placed Sumter resident who was mute and severely disturbed.

My routine with Gabe ever so gradually turned into a connection. I said "Hi, Gabe." And he echoed "Hi, Gabe." He began following me at a distance as I made my way on foot to the residence cabins I needed to visit. He would sit cross-legged in the dirt nearby rocking, and then follow me back to my office. If I had too much to carry, I would wordlessly hand some to him and he would carry part of my load as he trailed me around. One morning when I said, "Hi, Gabe, how are you?" he responded "Hi, Gabe...Fine, I'm fine." This was to my knowledge the first non-echoed response anyone had gotten from this mysterious man.

Gabe helped me carry my various loads—books, reinforcers, stimulators—from one end of the Sumter campus to the other. He had been given and he accepted small tasks to complete while he waited for me. He had begun to make eye contact as he spoke. In time, we found that he knew his first name but not his last. When asked about family, he merely waved his arms dismissively.

Gabe spent long spans of time sitting and staring up at the sky. Occasionally, I would sit down next to him on the ground and share his silent musing of the heavens. Lucy, my extraordinarily talented and intuitive occupational therapist friend, told me that Gabe seemed to be able to do jobs considerably above his supposed level of intellect. We collectively began to wonder if he was mentally impaired or devastatingly traumatized by the events in his life. All of us, in all three therapies—speech, occupational and physical—enjoyed our new mascot and friend. Apparently he grew very attached to all of us as well. His cottage staff reported that he would hurriedly eat breakfast and dart out the door to run-walk in the direction of the therapy buildings.

One incident cemented my relationship with Gabe. I was working at my desk in the speech office when I heard yelling outside. A large, male counselor was pulling Gabe off the ground—dragging, really—and scolding him. Gabe was skinny and about half the counselor's size. I demanded that the counselor get go of "my resident." We played tug-of-war with Gabe until the big man surrendered him to me. I brought Gabe inside, sat him down near me, and tried to calm him down. After a while of screaming, Gabe sat, staring ahead and rocking. "Ok, now, ok now, Gabe ok now," he assured me. I walked him to his cottage and into the care of his house staff.

Gabe taught me the value of respect. I believe it was because I treated him as a fellow human being that he had begun to interact. In the months before Sumter was due to close, and in the weeks before he was to be moved, I felt that I needed to prepare my new friend for our goodbyes. I showed him Sumter on the map and traced the way up to his group home. Gabe would nod and say, "Gabe move. Lydia. Gabe group home." Gabe left Sumter for placement in one of the group homes that started to accept the residents of Sumter soon after I left. Gabe was now a desirable and helpful housemate. He said goodbye to Lucy. He said goodbye to Ellen. He hugged me for a long time. He took the hand-drawn map with the traced path to his new home that I had left on my desk and said, "Lydia. No group home. Gabe group home."

One Christmas

My husband, Skip, plays with miniature trains. Originally bought with the purpose of engaging with his stepson, Ian, the hobby got out of hand and took over our living room, our backyard, and our vacations. He has a garden railroad and a table-top modular railroad. These are G-scale or large-scale trains complete with inch-and-a-half tall people populating large-scale houses, factories, and stations. Fascinated with Sumter and wishing to entertain my residents, Skip got permission to set up his two loops of track and three buildings in a picnic pavilion in the middle of the Sumter campus. Cottage caregivers crossed the generously treed park-like area between Sumter's boulevards to take their charges to and from workshops, cottages, or clinic. As they passed the pavilion, they were allowed to stop and watch the trains. The trains were a destination for other specific residents—a way to entertain bored, rambunctious folks. Without exception, all of the residents were fascinated with the trains and stood or sat mesmerized as the trains made the loops supposedly on their own. Several of the men would "whoop" when the train whistle blew. The rockers would stand quietly and rock as they watched. The autistics generally flapped their fingers while swaying from one foot to the other.

One resident's mother was visiting him for the holiday. They walked to the pavilion together to watch the trains. He watched wide-eyed for moments then threw back his head and let out a loud, "Woo Woo!" in imitation of the little train's whistle. His mom, happy tears in her eyes, informed us that she had never heard her son's voice before.

One young well-groomed man, Clarence, lagged behind his cottage group and took a seat next to Skip. He was a pleasant, slight man in his early '20s who was verbal and especially polite.

"Skip, sir, may I please see the trains again?"

"Please sir, may I hold the controls?" he'd say in true Southern style.

Clarence stayed in the pavilion alone with Skip for a long while, apparently not missed by his caregiver.

A therapist came by, saw Clarence, and asked Skip, "Are you okay? Is it all right if he is here?" Skip had begun to think of Clarence as a staff member or a relative who had come to visit. Clarence was definitely not run-of-the-mill Sumter material. Skip was puzzled as to why this young man stayed and why people questioned his own safety. When my obligations finished, I joined Skip in the afternoon to keep him company and observe the enjoyment the residents demonstrated in the trains. I greeted Clarence, also surprised he was there unaccompanied.

Skip approached me, leaving the train controls in the care of Clarence and queried, "What a nice young man! Why isn't he at home with his family for the holidays?"

After I finished laughing, I told Skip, "He has no family. He killed them!"

Clarence was a newcomer to Sumter; he had nowhere else to go, was adjudged not of sound mind or whatever legal stuff went on, and because he was also autistic (autistoid?) was plopped in Sumter. It seemed that the newborn baby twins were just making too much noise, crying all the time—so he set his mobile home on fire. In addition to his two siblings, his parents were trapped in the blaze and burned to death. So Sumter got another resident.

Everyone who paused to see if Clarence would implode when the train whistle blew was disappointed. Months of Sensory Integration helped Clarence stay calm. Either that or he ran out of crying infants. Or matches.

A Whole Different Ballgame

Admittedly, I had been fortunate to experience a wealth of different and exotic cases in my career. I don't think for a moment I could have stayed in one position year after year, seeing only stroke patients, voice patients, or pediatric patients. Choosing to be contracted to a variety of facilities exposed me to ventilator-dependent individuals, abused children lying in coma after horrific beatings, prematurely born infants who needed to be trained to suckle, psychiatric patients at the state hospital who were drug dependent on substances which rendered them incomprehensible, and a variety of neurologically impaired adults. This was my "home base." In the ever-changing world of Medicare regulations and the demographics of South Florida in the twenty-six years I'd lived there, and then as a newcomer to South Carolina, I tried to keep up with the needs of my profession.

I learned how to handle kids, expanding my position in an acute care hospital from neurologically involved adults to outpatient "birth-through-three-year-old" children. I grew attached to many of my little patients, but never quite felt at home. Just before I left South Florida, I had worked at Baby House, a group home for the profoundly retarded birth-to-five population. I did a lot of "passive stimulation" on gums and cheeks in an effort to tweak out a mere glimmer of movement that could be harvested for sound.

These children were aware of me only as a source of warmth or aggravation, and they either allowed hugs or they physically attacked me. It was not the job for me. I was warned that the people I'd be working with at Sumter were "Baby House grown-ups" and that they would "just drool all over you." Yuck. I had a good reason for taking on such an adventure. I needed a job in my new state. The hospital work that was my first love was not interviewing. I'd give this Sumter job a try.

My supervisor, mentor, and forever friend, Ellen, threw me a softball for my first evaluation. I grabbed up my traveling kit of test materials, paper, pen, and then went to meet Keith. Keith was verbal, though barely understandable, but his scant vocabulary allowed me to grab hold and actually make a speech and language diagnosis. I accepted this relatively easy case. The old insurance rule of get-in-and-get-it-done-quickly had kicked in. I nailed Keith and his deficits down on paper in a little over one hour. I marched back to Ellen very satisfied with myself and handed her the typed evaluation.

She read it, smiled and said, "Why are you in such a hurry? Take your time with Keith, get to know him."

Huh? I thought. This was different. I wasn't on a deadline? There was no pressure to get it done quickly? I was very confused.

"What do you mean, *get to know him*? What is it I'm supposed to do?" I asked.

Ellen thought a while, and then responded, "All these people here, they are not 'patients.' We refer to them as 'residents.' Pretend you are their Mom and that they are all your children. Then, do what is best for them."

Indeed, Sumter required paperwork but the documentation was different: a pages-long study of all of the interpretable facets of the resident's skills, likes (reinforcers), dislikes (non-negotiables), pet peeves (whatever set them off) as well as characteristics of their speech, language, and eating behaviors. Along with the luxury of time spent with each, what contrasted the most with my previous life was team treatment. Every resident was picked over and cared for by a team of doctors on site, neuropsychologists, behavioral psychologists, psychiatrists, physical therapists, occupational therapists, dietitians, cottage caregivers and me, one of a team of speech-language pathologists.

We met in weekly meetings or meetings set up emergently to discuss routine or immediate problems. In addition to all the people listed above, Sumter had a cadre of administrators, interpreters of ever-changing legislation, state auditors, federal auditors and more. We knew when the big wigs were due to visit because the grass would get cut and the trees pruned. The campus would be clean and tidy for a short while. Many times I wished my elderly stroke patients would get a smidgen of the resources the Sumter residents got.

When I figured out I could actually take the time to study my new treatment population, my anxiety ceased. I went about "learning" Sumter the same way I applied myself to anything I was motivated to know, immersion. I immersed myself in everything Sumter. I began by visiting the cottages assigned to me. Ellen divided the caseload by assigning each of the four of us several cottages, each housing twelve residents.

Depending on the behavior, capacity, or independence level of the resident, each was given a bed in a single, double, or dormitory-style room. Each cottage had communal bath, toilet and wash rooms. Each cottage had a great room with an adjoining pass-through kitchen, dining area, and TV room.

My first cottage housed men who were ambulatory and relatively independent. They all had jobs in the paper-recycling workshop—a relatively easy job of unfolding newspaper and fitting it into a frame. The even-edged newspaper would then be rolled and placed on large shelves to be taken to a recycling center.

I entered the house, introduced myself to the house staff of two to four men and women. Some of these caregivers had been in their jobs for decades, and they'd actually raised the residents from the time the residents were children when the State of South Carolina had placed them at Sumter Center, then a facility for the institutionalization of the profoundly retarded. When I entered the scene in 2000, the residents ranged from a newly-placed twenty-year-old forsaken by his parents when he became dangerously physically abusive, to wheelchair-bound folks in their 60s and 70s. Not knowing how else to proceed, I took the only seat available on the cottage couch, between two middle-aged men. I attempted to engage but was ignored.

Other men in the cottage ambled over to stare at me or reach out and touch my hair but basically we three just sat on the couch bonding. The caregivers stole glances at me and I smiled back at them with all the confidence of knowing exactly what I was doing—which, of course, I did not. But it eventually worked for me as it was the best way for me to see my clients in their natural habitat.

As I sat in one house with my new best friends, Ellen happened to come to the door. She looked very surprised to see me there, not standing apart and taking notes or talking to caregivers but looking for all the world like my new charges—right smack in the middle of the napping, rocking, slobbering, nose picking, masturbating household. Ellen later laughed and said she had never considered hobnobbing with the residents as a way to learn them, but she didn't have to. Unlike me, this population was her life's work and she knew this population better than anyone. When I came up with an insight about my residents, I ran it past Ellen.

Occasionally she would look at me in wonder: "Wow! I never thought of that."

I would answer, not at all or, maybe a little disingenuously, "I feel…adequate." It felt good. To be adequate, to have insights, to be listened to, to be welcomed. It felt damned good.

There were new things for me to learn in every corner of Sumter starting with what a resident expected of me. To some, I was very much a part of the environment. My hand would be placed on someone's arm and moved to scratch or stroke, so often I felt like a tool rather than a person. To others, I was a disseminator of treats: "cokecokecoke" was a greeting Mary offered upon seeing me. I was a backscratcher. I was a cushion. I was a dance partner. I was someone to hug. I was justifiably proud when I figured out what my charges wanted. Most residents taught me to be patient and just observe, hang out, and watch.

In Jail

One fascinating area of the Sumter Center campus was the chain-link quad a-hundred yards directly behind our therapy buildings. Within the twelve-foot fence were two cottages, which looked much the same as the others, and were surrounded by a scraggly lawn and an unkempt basketball court. This was the Pathway Program. The quad housed developmentally delayed male prisoners—those determined "incompetent to proceed" in criminal court. They were found guilty and had to be housed somewhere on state property so they were placed at Sumter. For all intents, these men were doubly imprisoned within the locked-tight community walls and the chain link of their quad. I don't know if these guys were any more or less a threat to anyone. One of my prisoner residents had been convicted of armed robbery of a uniformed cop. Another had been imprisoned for exposing himself, a "crime" many of the residents perpetrated daily within the hallowed community walls outside the chain link.

Ellen assigned two of the prisoners to me for language stimulation. They had set appointments and a burly caregiver/guard brought them to our speech building. The guards then had to sit (bored, no doubt) while we provided the state-financed language lesson. I found my two guys to be charming, grateful for our attention, and motivated to improve. Without too much trouble, I discovered both of them enjoyed Coke. (Was the whole community addicted to Coca Cola?) One of our lessons involved reading, a skill neither of them had. But I was determined to enlighten my two charges on the finer points of finding a 'men's room' on their own or paying attention to a 'don't walk' sign, among other helpful hints on negotiating the outside world, should they ever be reintroduced into society.

One of my favorite lessons was "Scavenger Hunt." It did not involve much sit-down-and-listen since neither of the boys could do so. I made up clues I had written and drawn on separate pieces of paper, which I hid around the speech building: under desks, taped to a wall, behind the bookcase, etc. Each piece of paper was a clue to the next piece of paper. The drawn pictures or diagrams were combined with one of two large print upper or lower case words, which could easily be read with the help of the drawing.

When the two guys put their heads together trying to interpret each clue, all of us had stopped to watch. They were determined and sometimes stumbled too impulsively going in all the wrong directions, waiting to be told "you're getting warmer" or "no, now you're getting colder." Some of the humor for me was that these were convicted "armed and dangerous" criminals working their tails off to get their can of Coke at the end of the hunt.

One of the guys, Walt, ran the community car detailing shop in an effort for the State to teach him work skills, and to earn the prisoners some money. At first, the worker-bees like myself were apprehensive about entrusting our cars to less-than-intellectually- sterling prisoners who lacked a sense of property boundaries. In time, the work was so good, and the cars were so immaculate, that Walt had a steady line of employees and state cars lined up twice each week to be detailed. My coins stayed in the change hole. My CDs remained in their cases and my other valuables were sometimes cleaned up and shined, too, much to my amazement.

When Sumter Center was officially closed, these cons did not get moved like the rest of the residents to lovely neighborhood group homes. They either stayed within their fenced in quad as the State of South Carolina worked to seek out other uses for the huge property, or were moved to another state facility, which was permitted to house these double prisoners.

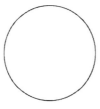

Isadora

Isadora was, without a doubt, one of the more challenging cases that Ellen had given to me. In time she would open my head and my heart in ways no other human ever had. Ellen had told me Isadora would be very difficult to look at, and that her situation was very difficult to accept. I was given directions to the newspaper recycling building and prepared myself. Despite the ghastly description and warnings of distress that I had been given, I had to search the room carefully for Isadora. I expected much worse. She was a spare figure, not easily noticed. Isadora was born with Treacher-Collins Syndrome. She presented with a cleft face—no nose, just a hole; flat, virtually absent cheek bones; and bug-like eyes on either side of her head with the crevasse ending at her lower lip. No teeth graced her smile but I could tell when she was smiling, the way one could see a favored pup smiling—by the way it held its head, and the subtle curve of its lip. Isadora smiled.

Many hours of plastic reconstruction formed a nose (of sorts) which could breathe, and had brought her eyes closer together. One eye was blind, so the lack of congruence didn't affect the seeing eye. Her mouth could eat and breathe, but could not speak. But she smiled! I asked her work supervisor to get her for me, and I told both of them that I would be taking Isadora to speech therapy. Isadora arose, cocked her head to better see me, and then scanned my body almost touching from top to bottom to get familiar with the way I looked—and maybe with the way I smelled. She held out her arm to me to be led.

I let go of her after a few moments during the short walk to the speech building, but it was enough time for her to dance away from me, skipping and arabesqueing way ahead of me. When she skipped along, which I learned she often did in her gaiety, she was radiant and anything but deformed. I assumed she could not see well, would trip, would get hurt, so I ran to her to grab her again. She docilely came along. Inside my

157

office, Stacy, my officemate and Isadora's former speech therapist, brought me up to snuff on Isadora's progress to date.

Stacy had been working on eating and swallowing with Isadora. I did not want to cover old tracks but wished to forge onward. I did a very cursory oral motor examination of my new resident, which was very cursory since Isadora absolutely did not wish anyone rummaging around in her mouth. She had no mandible, which allowed her mouth to hang from the cheeks. She kept her mouth open to help her breathe. I recall a tongue, which had limited movement. She would not allow a look beyond for me to see her palate, if there was one. I spoke to her hoping that she would understand me, but she did not seem to. She got out of the chair I indicated she sit in to instead walk around the room, touching whatever she came across. After bending to see objects on tabletops, she selected one, put it next to the left side of her head and flicked it. If flicking made a high-pitched tinkly noise, she held on to the object. If not, it was put back and forgotten. The item making the loudest tinkly noise was kept. She would then find the door and leave with her find.

This happened so often, I knew to hide things I didn't want to lose, or simply go later to her cottage and retrieve my stuff from her room. In her cottage, I sat in a quiet (and not so quiet) place and observed Isadora with her housemates, women of middle age and younger (Isadora was to turn thirty soon), who were ambulatory and healthy. Mealtime came and the caregiver yelled, "Isadora!" To my amazement, Isadora responded. I did not think she could hear since she had no ear holes. No ears, no hearing, I thought, but foolish me. I had forgotten my long ago audiology classes, which told of vibratory hearing—sound waves vibrating on the skull transformed into sound by the inner ear.

Isadora was handed silverware with which she deftly set the cottage tables; she was very useful. Mealtime afforded me the opportunity to see how Isadora received nourishment. Her plate was filled with pureed food: food the others were eating was blended for Isadora. She had no teeth, but managed to get food swallowed by pushing the food as far into her mouth with the spoon then mashing the puree with her tongue on the top of her oral cavity, eventually getting most of it to the back. She was not always successful and food dripped out her lips. She had a special cup that allowed her to pour liquids from a spout into her mouth without much mess. After speaking to Isadora's caregivers about her eating, I was satisfied that there was nothing I could do for her to make eating any easier: she was making the most of what she had.

I became more interested in Isadora's achievements, her ability to get around and dress herself, feed herself and even hold down cottage chores and a workshop job. I decided to immerse myself in Isadora-ness.

I had gotten so used to Isadora after months of treating her, observing her, and keeping her company, that I didn't see her anymore; she became just Isadora. A typical day went like this: I show up at her cottage. Without my beckoning her, she stands as I enter and approaches. She gives me her top-to-bottom look-and-sniff, then turns her long, tapered hands palm-down and hits the sides of her hands together before grabbing my hands. I don't know what it means. She pulls me out the door and drags me running and skipping.

I was told she had gone to special education schools, two of the best in the area, and learned how to communicate with her hands. But I don't know her language and she can't speak mine. She doesn't seem to care where we go; she leads, pulls me along, and randomly walks or runs with me in tow. By her posture and her skipping and the burbly sound from her throat, I postulate that she is happy. I consider that the curious banging of her hands before she pulls me means, "together." I feel giddy because I have solved one of her mysteries—or at least just a small part of her mystery.

As I watch her in my office going through her ritual of flicking objects near her head, I give her things that make louder sound when flicked. Her favorite was a musical triangle and its metal stick. Isadora is sent into raptures with this new toy and bangs away metal to metal, dancing around the room. I bring her into the sensory lab and observe her while she explores the room. She crawls onto the vibration mat atop a futon with her triangle and stick, and she curls into a fetal position banging and rocking. I turn on the bed's vibration to full and she stills and begins to coo. She lays there for forever and I need to drag her off the mat. In subsequent sessions, I give Isadora all matter of vibrating items: vibrating cushy pillows, a hand held animal, which vibrates, a back massager. She tries to take each to her cottage and I let her until I find she enjoys the items for a while, and then dismantles each one.

I have found not one but two behavior reinforcers for Isadora. I could then set about teaching Isadora to better communicate by promising her vibration or noisy toys. Of course, it eventually occurred to me that she was addicted to vibration and that flicking objects to make "noise" was her way of making enough vibration to conduct through her skull so she could hear it. I discover by witnessing Isadora's obvious desperate sadness when I took away her vibration that this was not a reinforcer but a nonnegotiable—something Isadora *needed.* I guess it wouldn't be too strong a metaphor to say that relieving oneself when one feels bladder pain is a nonnegotiable. Having determined that Isadora desperately needed vibration to survive, I knew then it was immoral and unethical for me to use vibration as a reinforcer. I used her vibration mat in the S.I. room as her reinforcer, an 'extra' treat and provided her with other forms of vibration in her cottage when work is over to calm herself.

I didn't know how much Isadora was taught as a child. No one was certain how "retarded" Isadora was. I theorized that Isadora's gesture of knocking the sides of her hands together was a form of sign language. I was unfamiliar with American Sign Language, so could only guess that her gesture might have been learned at some point. If she had it in her to learn signs, then I should have been able to enhance her signs and make them useful to those she lived with at that time. And if she had it in her to learn signs, so could I.

Ellen had an ancient book the size of a huge coffee table book. It had generous pictures of hands signing and on the facing page, the line drawing of what the sign stood for. Twice weekly, I brought Isadora to my office or I went to her house before mealtime and we worked on her signs. I sat Isadora down and I showed her large, bold-lined drawings of a house and the hand posture. She showed me peaked fingers for "house." A table and its hand posture: she placed her palms down and away for "table." A spoon and its hand posture: she held an imaginary spoon to her lips. Isadora knew how to sign! We concentrated on ten everyday signs that I suspected she had once mastered but now used carelessly and vaguely.

When I spent time with her outside of these sessions, she didn't attend to my signing and made no attempt to sign to me anything besides down turned palms banging. Well, except once when I assumed she was irritated with me. She held an imaginary stick in her hands—snapped it in half, and then turned her back to me. But she didn't care about my signs. No progress was made after many sessions and I was getting frustrated. She knew frustration, I am sure, and had learned through many years to cope with her own emotions and those of others. She still got angry but it took a lot. Mostly she displayed boredom and inattention, especially at my feeble attempts to communicate with her.

With very impaired stroke victims, the very least I will work on is a reliable and universal way of indicating "yes" or "no" with head movements. I realized one day that Isadora didn't have a reliable "yes" or "no." Heck, she'd never communicated "yes" or "no" at all. She responded to suggestions, commands, or questions with an action of her own.

On one of our hands-together-hands-grasp-my-wrists-gallop-through-the-campus, I stopped Isadora and asked her a question that I knew she would say yes to: "Do you want to walk more?" Then I took her head and manually moved it up and down in a nod, all the while saying, "Yes! This is Yes!"

We galloped, galloped, and then stopped again.

"Isadora do you want to walk more?" My hands were on either side of her head again, moving it up and down: "Yes! This is Yes!"

We galloped and galloped some more (I'm not as young as I used to be). We stopped and I asked her again: "Isadora, do you want to walk more?"

This time she responded by taking *my* head in *her* hands. Yes! That was Isadora's yes.

Isadora amazed. With one sort-of-seeing-eye and no ear holes, she knew when I arrived at her home. I watched as she followed commands to, "Set the tables, Iz."

She would respond with dance steps when loud music was on. I asked Isadora's doctor for permission to do an audiological examination. I could do a cursory hearing screen in my office. For comprehensive hearing tests, she would have to be taken to an audiologist. I offered to accompany her. We were given an appointment at the audiology lab, and an official car and driver.

Isadora was a challenge to test. The audiology testing required that the subject be seated in a small soundproof booth facing a window. On the other side of the window were the controls and the tester. First, I sat in the sound-proof audiology booth with Isadora, rather than on the tester's side. She was visibly nervous, if not scared. She would not sit in the chair or face the window. We had to condition her with play therapy the way babies have their hearing tested. Isadora was too distracted and wanted to know all about this new environment. When her examiner and I tried firmness, her feelings had become hurt and she pouted and did nothing at all.

The test took a long, long time. Finally, through trial and error, the audiologist arrived at Isadora's functional hearing level. The audiologist decided that Isadora needed a bone conduction hearing aid, which uses vibration directly onto the skull. The oscillator was connected to one side of a headband. Wires connected the oscillator to a battery and amplifier on the opposite side of a headband. The oscillator was positioned as close to the temporal bone as was possible. Older models positioned the oscillator onto the forehead with wires leading to a clumsy, big battery pack in the person's pocket. The bones directed the vibration to the inner ear, which then would perceive and process the vibration into noise, voice, and even speech. Bone conduction hearing aids weren't as effective as ear channel hearing aids, but Isadora had no outer ear, no ear channels.

Isadora once had a bone conductor hearing aid, which she wore in her front pocket. It was a heavy thing—the size of a deck of playing cards, with wires snaking up to a curved wire worn around the back of her half-formed conch-shell of an earlobe. She continually had taken her bone conductor off to take it apart and see how it worked. Finally, her caregivers gave up and put the thing in a drawer, where it was forgotten.

Her audiologist and I pondered how to deliver the sound vibration. We decided Iz's hearing aid could be put onto a headband. Isadora's house staff occasionally plaited her hair and kept her hairdo neat with headbands, so headbands weren't strange nor exotic to Isadora. The headband positioned the oscillator so it sat pressed to her right mastoid process (bone behind ear). Her audiogram showed that her other inner ear picked up very little hearing, so the right side of her head was chosen for vibration to that side's inner ear.

Finally, Isadora's custom headband hearing aid was ready. Isadora and I commandeered another Sumter Center car and driver and eagerly went to pick up her new hearing aid. Any of the residents obtaining an impressive piece of technology like Isadora's hearing aid was no small thing for Sumter Center. A bunch of us—Iz's house moms, the therapists, a few psychologists and the Center's physician—turned up for Isadora's maiden voyage with her new hearing aid. We all had expected the likes of Bell's first phone call to Watson. But aside from looking around a bit more, Isadora hadn't indicated that her hearing was better or worse. Of course, we didn't have to raise our voices when asking her to do chores. I figured out after a time that what Isadora chose to hear, she heard and otherwise she flat out ignored you—just like the rest of us.

What really made our day was playing music for her when she had her headband on. Isadora danced and showed some pretty hip moves. She skipped around and looked for metal she could hit on metal to make tinkly sounds close to her headband amplifier. She really liked the now-louder, tinkly, high-pitched sounds. Isadora's dependence on vibration made keeping the headband on her head possible. Her hearing aid was a good, socially acceptable and socially-enhancing tool for her. It sat on her head and vibrated whenever the amplifier picked up sound. I think for the same reason one would douse a taco with habanero sauce, Isadora beat objects together near her amplifier to kick up the volume, so to speak, on her vibratory experience.

Isadora also demonstrated sensitivity to cold and a desire for heat. As we passed parked cars on a hot day, Isadora broke away from me and laid her cheek and upper body on the hood of the car, staying there for a minute or so. I imagined the car's surface to be burning hot but she seemed to enjoy the heat. She preferred a sweater, a jacket, or blanket on her most of the time. Each day I took Isadora out of work (to sort newspapers for recycling) and brought her into the sensory integration room. She headed straight for the vibrating bed and lay down. I handed her a blanket, which she snuggled around herself. This adult child lay on her side, faced the wall, and sighed a deep breath out, relaxing. I put a hand-held powerful massager for additional vibration in her exposed hand. She put the massager *against* her headband amplifier, and with a smile on her face, brought the blanket up over her head.

One person had worked at the center long enough to remember when Isadora arrived. It was April 13, 1998 and she was twenty-six and the veteran of countless surgeries and other traumas. Isadora was born in Aiken, South Carolina, down state from Sumter Center to a drug user. Rumor had it her mother, a street prostitute, chose to turn her birth-deformed daughter out onto the streets rather than to leave her alone in her apartment. Eventually, her mother handed Isadora over to the state, not wishing to be saddled with the endless medical procedures, or carry her on her appointed rounds. Isadora essentially spent her early years living in one institution after another, eventually landing in a facility for the insane.

Later, newspaper headlines would inform an unsuspecting public of the nightmares that disabled, institutionalized children survived. When Isadora was twenty-four, she ended up at an aunt's home in Anderson, South Carolina. From her aunt's, she went from place-to-place until she was admitted to a local hospital. She was diagnosed with "failure to thrive" and Sumter Center was chosen by the state as the best place for her.

Later, in 2001, Isadora didn't fit any "diagnosis." I marveled at the way labels such as "autistic" "retarded" "schizophrenic" "conduct disordered" each fit different behavior patterns. Other people, including some psychologists who worked within Sumter's gates, considered the residents to be big children, or big infants, depending on how concretely the residents related to their environment. These professionals were grounded, it seemed, in assuming that the residents were like the old, predictable lab animals, upon which they trained. Stimulus leads to response. Comfortable. Reliable. Reinforced behavior leads to changed behavior. My own conclusion was that infants and children were *normal* or more aptly, familiar people. They would mature and share a reality similar to our own. But our residents were adults, and being mature, would be expected to have grown to be independent and able to function on their own. They never did.

These adults had massive anxiety and coping dysfunctions: each required repetitive, tolerant one-on-one shaping in order to just share space with others. My residents had to be taught what was food, what was not food, and how to eat food. Residents' perceptions and reactions seemed out of kilter from the rest of us. The rest of US...the "general," bell-curve "average" public who share a common reality. Don't we trust that when we speak, others understand? That what we speak about, others have experienced? My residents seemed quite exotic from the folks familiar to me. Exotic brains perceive the world very differently than the rest of us: sounds, sights, touches are louder, softer or distorted; sometimes they are unbearable, sometimes they are a source of exquisite pleasure.

When a resident is removed from his familiar, and, therefore, safe environment, it is many times frightening, threatening, overwhelming. The terrain for them seems very different from the world the rest of us experience, and so are their actions. We understand just a little what role perception can contribute, and how devastating it can be when that perception is fractured.

I have entertained the thought that residents have been done a disservice putting them in the same frame of reference as the other people with whom the world is shared. These folks are "delayed" but will never catch up. The Diagnostic and Statistical Manual of Mental Disorders addresses developmental disorders as well as schizophrenia and autism as mental disorders; but as I got to know the residents of Sumter, and those similar to them in my outside world, I wondered if rather than damaged brains they could be considered something other. If we apply the societal "rules" to people who somehow fit on one of the Manual's Axes, they lose. If we make new rules, perhaps, then we wouldn't set the bar too high. Those with developmental delay who show autistoid or schizoid characteristics won't need to adapt behavior-warping, unsuccessful coping skills that set them even further apart from "us."

Perception—most formally classified by sight, sound, touch, smell, proprioception and kinesthesia—plays a significant role in the daily lives of humans. We see, hear, feel to sense threat and can protect ourselves. Humans have created tools to use to secure our own safety. We speak and communicate to secure our own safety. Beyond basic safety, we create and communicate to advance ourselves and for pleasure. Humans are hunters—we consider ourselves to be at the top of the food chain. We kill and eat other animals. We enjoy a certain amount of control over our environment. I wanted to learn more about the control my residents had acquired. I needed to understand my residents' natures.

I have enjoyed reading several of the works by Temple Grandin, who has autism. She has matured into a person who has come to an understanding of her own needs. She writes that through her own experiences she understands the nature of prey animals—specifically cows. I don't truly know if my insight had come from reading Ms. Grandin's books or whether I came to intuitive conclusions on my own. I do know that living closely with an animal I had wrapped my heart around has brought me closer to touching the experiences of the exotic people who lived in Sumter.

In adopting and committing to raising a pet pig, we needed to learn about pigs. We should not have assumed that pigs are like dogs, that raising a pig would be similar to raising a dog. At first we did assume Peg shared nature with our two dogs, Havoc and Murphy. After all, when we adopted Peg, she was too early away from her mother. Two weeks old and hand-fed by one of us, she had no idea she was a pig. A human, perhaps—another dog, certainly. Three humans and two dogs were all Peg knew. Yet raising her in our home, being in proximity to her, handling and loving her, we came to know that pigs are a totally different animal. I had begun to see the usefulness of learning my pig the way I was beginning to know my Sumter residents. My Sumter residents were likewise a totally different kind of animal.

Temple Grandin had her cows and Lydia had her pig.

Millennium Pig

Pigs are prey. That's the way they are built inside and out. Their eyesight is poor, and they are said to be color blind and have poor depth perception which results in an extreme sensitivity to contrasts. Peggy the pig startled easily at shadows. Noises frightened her. Pigs can develop a fondness for routine and for their own turf, minimizing surprises that have the potential to injure or kill. To build rapport with Peggy, I needed to be very patient and spend time observing her. My resident, Gabe's lesson to me also came into play—I needed to respect Peggy's pigness.

My family and I read any and all books we could find on raising a miniature pig. We learned health-related information and very basic characteristics, and also discovered that potbellied pigs were very much in vogue. Early on, we took one book's advice and bought a harness for Peg. She had quickly learned to pee in a designated place inside the house. She learned to walk with us on her harness just as quickly. It wasn't instantaneous; it took some perseverance, but after days of squealing and balking, she found the harness quite to her liking, especially since it allowed her to go on walks around the neighborhood so that she could see things outside of the house. Our neighbors quickly got used to the two or three of us walking the two dogs and one pig down the street.

When Peg was bad, and she was bad in big ways (such as when she uprooted expensive landscaping or broke out of her pen), we needed to shape her behavior. She did not take to being threatened with a stick or a palm. She got wacko and attacked us. This is amusing when a pig is small, but not so funny when a pig weighs as much as you do. Mama pigs discipline their piglets by pushing them. Shoving gets their attention quickly since they don't want to lose their balance walking on their dainty high-heeled hooves. Shoving helped me discipline and train Peg quite easily.

Peg eventually began to share the dog pen with the two dogs, believing for all-the-world that she was a smart dog and they were two stupid, uglier dogs. When the dogs ran to the fence and barked, so did Peg. When treats were handed out, all three sat and waited. All three had access to the backyard, but Peggy learned how to open the door and let herself into the house on hot days. Our downstairs screen door to the backyard was left unlocked. The catch that held the door closed was removed. A wooden triangle was screwed on to the bottom of the door. Peg could fit her nose in the triangle and draw open the screen door; and she went a step further.

We came home one day to find the fridge we kept in the basement standing open and everything that had been inside it all over the basement floor. Peg had released the door with her nose and had drunk all of the beer and soda in the fridge. She picked up each can, pierced the can with her sharp front teeth, tipped her head back, and let the liquid flow onto her head and into her mouth.

When she had stolen a sweet potato from me intending on playing keep away, she discovered she liked eating them and continued to try to steal foods she liked. One day, we left her alone with the run of the house. When we arrived home we couldn't find her. We looked all over calling, "Peg-gy!, Peg-gy!" She was nowhere. Scratching our heads in the middle of the kitchen, we heard a single grunt. She had pushed the louvered door into the pantry, and had gotten into the cooking wine bottles stored on the floor. She unscrewed the bottles and finished off all the wine. But the louvered door closed behind her and she was trapped in the pantry. When we found her and let her out, a very tipsy little pig staggered around the house and eventually fell asleep in the dining room.

When Peg was little and we still lived in Florida, she perfected climbing into our SUV. We built a ramp. By placing pieces of apple along the length of the ramp, we taught Peggy to walk up the ramp and into the SUV so that we could take her and the dogs to parks for a change of pace. One of our favorite parks was an oak-forested beauty with acres of grassy meadows. We had taken all three off their leashes and let them gambol. All three sniffed around, ran together and seemed to enjoy one another's company. When we called them back, only the pig obeyed. This got the attention of a secret observer who admitted that he watched our family whenever we came to the park.

Dennis was in the business of procuring animals for movies and special events, and he had a deep appreciation of animal training. He approached us to ask if we would consider renting Peggy to him for photo shoots or other opportunities that turned up. We agreed, but made clear that she was special and that one of us would have to go with her or bring her to the shoots. Dennis called some time later and asked us to drive Peg to his place, where he would transport her in his horse trailer like a common animal to a photo shoot in the Florida keys that weekend. Nope, we said, we will take her. Dennis promised good money, but I couldn't go because of work. My son, Ian, who was eighteen at the time, refused to go along; there were better things to do than babysit a pig. So my husband, Skip, took Peg by himself. He called Ian from the photo shoot to say, "You're going to regret not coming with me, the models are all naked!" Dennis hadn't informed us that the photo shoot was for Abercrombie and Fitch. The set was populated by gorgeous, nude, young, male and female models.

Dennis made that trip to The Keys financially worthwhile. He next secured a job for Peggy as the star of a CSI episode, which would spin off *CSI: Miami* from the original *CSI:Crime Scene Investigation* that took place in Las Vegas. Peg's part in the filming would take place one month after the Abercrombie and Fitch shoot. I was not going to stay away from this job. Skip and I drove our starlet Peggy to the set, in a remote part of Homestead, Florida.

Peggy was assigned a "butler" who dragged around a water hose, so she had mud to wallow in as needed. It was April and hot. Pigs don't sweat (and people don't "sweat like a pig"). Pigs regulate their body temperature by wallowing. It was hot enough that day that I was tempted to join her. Dennis told the producers that Peg liked her beer. So, naturally, her favorite beer was provided as well as some chicken and beef jerky that the production company figured she might appreciate. We humans trailed along, butler-less without benefit of water, beer, or jerky.

The storyline of the show had the Las Vegas police chief murdered and displayed on his dining table trussed up with an apple in his mouth (like a pig, get it?). His wife and daughter were kidnapped and brought to Miami. David Caruso, the star of *CSI:Miami* was to search high and low for the child, and then have a peacock squawk to get his attention. He was to follow the peacock and find the girl in the

Everglades. Dennis, Peg's agent and manager, was the production's animal procurer. He reminded the producer of one detail—peacocks aren't found in the Everglades, and it wasn't likely that one would be wandering around to opportunistically make noise to attract attention. Besides, Dennis had a pig, not a peacock. He explained to the producers that a wild boar would be more to the point and would better fit into the script. Hence, Peggy. So, Peggy was to do her walk on, which was actually a scuttle across a dusty gravel road. The script had her grunt and continue going into the glades. Caruso would follow and find Peggy-the-heinous-wild-boar standing next to the little kidnapped girl. Not likely in real life. Besides, I think wild boars eat little children. Maybe not. So, the story was slightly rewritten to have Peg grunt and poop in the gravel road so that Caruso could find the girl's barrette lying in the pig poop. Peg's walk-on was a hit. Through the years, Peggy earned her money and her beer.

Still-little Peggy was used to being carted around South Florida in the back seat of our SUV as long as the trip was short. Anything longer than an hour, for instance, and Peggy made retching noises. As 2002—and time to leave South Florida—grew closer, we had to plan on transporting our two-year-old, hundred-pound pig to South Carolina. We were looking at over twelve hours with frequent stops to get Peggy to Greenville, South Carolina. The possibility that Peg might get car sick was considered—we weren't looking forward to her retching, nausea, and vomiting.

Halloween, 2002: The moving vans were packed and on their way. Skip and I dropped the dogs at his parents' house. We decided that the best strategy would be to take turns driving while the other tended to Peg. Our vet had come to the house and had given Peg an injection of a strong sedative combined with an anti-nausea medication. We felt sure that since she was medicated for nausea and sedated, she would be asleep in a heartbeat. So we crated our cat and loaded Peg, the crated cat and our luggage into the SUV. In preparation for our trip with Peggy, we lined the back of our SUV with layers of absorbent blankets and toweling sandwiched between plastic. We were confident that if Peg had an accident, the top layer could be rolled up and bagged, leaving her the next layer. This trip would be a relaxing piece of cake. Skip, Lydia, cat, and Peg were ready to make the journey.

About an hour later, before we had even left the county, Peggy wide-awake and belligerent, had become car sick. She grew anxious and tried to push her way into the front seat. We stopped several times to calm our pig down. Pig was beyond retching—her vomiting was torrential and nonstop. We jettisoned multiple layers of plastic and toweling along the side of the highway for the sodden, stinking mess and nowhere to dispose of it. The inadequate garbage bags we brought had quickly and woefully maxed out. Then we had to somehow secure the front seat so Peg couldn't get through. Abandoned to the rear of the SUV, Peg violently flipped the cat's crate around. Poor cat wasn't going to make it to South Carolina. Skip was able to ignore Peg's screams and the sounds of her throwing up and peeing in order to concentrate on driving. I agreed to climb in the back with Peg and the cat and keep order. The stench was unreal. I sat in damp urine and vomit-encrusted splendor. Mile after exhausting mile, Peg screamed and spewed. Eventually, she grew quieter and finally fell asleep. In Columbia, South Carolina.

Peg is now thirteen years old. She's still a "teacup," but a teacup weighing in at three-hundred-pounds. She lives in a room in our walk-out basement. She independently opens and closes the door to walk around in her own fenced-in, protected, shady backyard. Peg has become arthritic and doesn't wander much except when there is good stuff to harvest from my garden, or to eat acorns from our forest of oak trees.

She has a language we can readily understand. When she spots us, she approaches, pulls back her open mouth a bit which looks for all the world like a smile and huffs "ha-ha-ha-ha." There's no question this says: "Hello! I love you!" A quick half-turn and a "bonk" with her head to my leg means Peg's content and wants to play. A low rumbling signifies discontent or: "Get lost!" A high-pitched continuous siren tells me: "Please spend time with me, I miss you, Mom!" She accompanies this siren-pitch with a flip onto her side and waits to have her tummy rubbed. Our pig keeps track of our presence with intermittent "aaa-ee!" noise, which she appreciates having returned. If her routine is interrupted (naptime or dinner without due warning), I expect a frontal head butt— and a large contusion. Special moments between us are the times she croons and moans and squeaks when she is petted. Her eyes close and she lies still, stretching her legs and arching her neck backward. Alertness is evident with a sudden stop, eyes wide and scanning, ears straight up.

It was difficult at first figuring out when to scold Peggy or just appreciate that Peggy was doing something in her nature, but what seemed like bad behavior to us. For example she had a habit of breaking off branches from bushes and dragging them to her area of the yard. Pigs build nests in the wild as protection from the cold and to raise their young. This is hard-wired into pigs. Our Peg was neutered. She had never been exposed to the wild or to other pigs. And she didn't need a nest to raise babies. Peggy sleeps in the house on her very own couch covered in blankets. Yet our Pegasus built nests out of our azaleas. Nothing in the form of reasoning or punishment broke her out of destroying our landscaping. As I learned to do with my residents in Sumter, I sat and observed; we eventually got pig-smart. We bought our pig her very own bale of straw, and she pulled the straw apart and built her nest. Things between us humans and pig got much better.

We needed to understand Peg's need to be secure before she could attend to our requests to "Come!" "Sit!" "Back off!" or "Push the ball, Peg." Intuition told me to apply my S.I. techniques to my now-adult pig, Peg. I was learning so much from my good friends at Sumter. First, ensure security. Foster trust and reliability. Accustom to proximity and touch. Reinforce desirable behavior; ignore or use time out for negative behavior. Emphasize gently who is boss. Provide reliable, respectful, and loving behavior to pig and pig will return same.

As a speech language pathologist, I added another "language" to my repertoire: I speak English, a little Russian, Spanglish, aphasic, and pig.

Isadora, redux

Peggy taught me a lot. Isadora taught me much more; she illustrated just how much practical work one can usefully do with vast handicaps. Without benefit of adequate hearing or good vision and apparently diminished intellect, this amazing woman set the table for meals, cleaned the tables off later, and stacked the dishes and silverware in the dishwasher. She knew every inch of her community and could negotiate her way to work and home again by herself. She earned a living by processing newspapers for recycling. I think she was capable of so much more but, unfortunately, Isadora was also lazy. But was Isadora intelligent? We will never know absolutely because she was untestable by our standards. We would have to judge her by her actions and accomplishments. But first we would have to break her code.

Just as she *chose* to ignore us when she didn't *want* to hear us, she could queer an intelligence test with behavior not readily familiar and therefore not expected. It was very easy for folks throughout Isadora's life to label her "retarded." My feeling is that with the obstacles Iz had to surmount, the coping mechanisms she had to adapt, and the seeming instincts for life this woman had, she was anything but retarded.

One day while I was drawing symbols for her to sign, I impulsively handed her the marker and told her to write her name, so she did. *Good God,* I thought, *there is no end to Isadora's marvels. What else can she communicate?* But alas, she gave me nothing beyond letters in an organized alphabet and a series of numbers—she did not write other words to express herself. Maybe she knew how, maybe not. Maybe I could have taught her meaningful written words, maybe not. It seemed to me Isadora was just not interested.

After she successfully got us to actually do something, to accompany her on her gallops through the community, she began to sign more, in Isadora fashion. We weren't stupid dolts to her anymore once we began to understand her signs. Maybe she felt hopeful that we would make the effort to learn more of her signs. Maybe she took it for granted we already understood her signs. I wanted to help her to succeed with her communication, so I took a cue from Peggy. I couldn't speak "Pig" unless I knew the language. Instead of teaching Isadora, I taught her caregivers. Stacie, Ellen, Nadja and I (Sumter's Speech Department) took endless digital photographs of Isadora signing. We showed her pictures and clicked when she signed. Most of her signing looked the same but was quirky enough to be recognizable as meaning something specific.

After many, many photographs labeled with situations (peaked hands = house; two fingers on brow = tired, etc.), we picked the signs that were clearly and reliably associated with a concept or thing. We paired the concept with the photo of Isadora doing the sign her way. I made a picture book with these pictures of Isadora signing. Instead of doing therapy directly with Isadora, I conditioned her caregivers. I taught them what Isadora means when she signs. I knew this method was successful when, on one visit to her cottage, a staff member approached me with exuberance and amazement: "Isadora wanted the music turned on! She likes music! She *told* me!"

The state of South Carolina had decided to close Sumter Center and place all the residents in various group homes in neighborhoods. As it came time for Sumter Center to be closed, I worried about Isadora's fate. I had become very attached. I loved her. I will never have any idea if she reciprocated but she knew me, accepted me. I spoke to her state guardians about adoption. My son was off to university and we were just the two of us. We would find a place with us for Isadora. Isadora's Sumter cottage caregiver was planning on opening a group home on the coast for a select group of ladies from her cottage. She wanted Isadora to stay with her. She cared for and was familiar with Isadora: she should stay with her friends. While I was planning a return to hospital work, Ellen took the contract with the state to provide speech pathology services to a number of group homes statewide. She promised to stay in touch and send me news of Isadora's life. One of Ellen's emails, dated August 2006, read:

I still visit Isadora's home. I am teaching Isadora to sew. We started with a felt heart, which she sewed with a plastic needle and yarn, carefully feeling with her thumb to find out where the next hole was. She loves it! We have started on a teddy bear. We also tried a potting wheel a few weeks ago. Took her to a petting zoo— that was interesting! She continues to be a joy.

LTACH

In the eighties and nineties, I worked in an acute care hospital that leased space to a private corporation specializing in ventilator-dependent patients. I got to know my way around a ventilator, learned about tracheostomy, researched speaking valves and basically got a sample of just how sick people can become.

The Federal regulations in the mid-nineties, specifically the Balanced Budget Act of 1997, brought about many changes in healthcare. Acute care hospitals, the full-service institutions with emergency rooms, surgery suites and many beds, no longer found it profitable to keep patients after they were either medically stable or when they needed more time to become medically stable. The next rung of the healthcare ladder was post-acute care in a transitional care unit of the hospital, in a rehabilitation hospital, or in an extended care facility. For those in the ICUs too unstable to go home, or to any of the options listed above, another choice was made available. LTACH stands for long-term acute care hospital. Medically complex patients are transferred to a free-standing or hospital-within-a-hospital LTACH for about one month to receive the specialized, intensive care offered.

Sumter Center closed its doors forever in 2004. Jobless, the offer of employment in a once familiar venue was wonderful to me. A number of years had gone by and I needed to hone some long-neglected skills. Also, LTACHs had grown in sophistication and required all staff to undergo rigorous continuous training to keep up with the demands of working with chronically complex medical anomalies. I salivated at the challenge.

Chronic critical illness was a new concept for me, now in my second half-century of life and in the medical field for more than thirty years. I will try and explain this entity in my own words: If a person finds herself in an intensive care unit, it's usually because of traumatic injury, overwhelming infection, or other life-threatening condition. The ICU provides constant monitoring and comprehensive care. The biological changes that occur with a life-threatening episode are familiar to us all: fight-or-flight. The body rallies to defeat whatever *dis-ease* is menacing it. All of the body's "soldiers" get involved: the sympathetic nervous system, the immune system and the adrenal-endocrine system join forces to keep the heart pumping and keep the organs working. This fight-or-flight response was never meant to be long-term, and after a while, the body experiences multi-organ system dysfunction, commonly known as chronic critical illness syndrome.

LTACH patients are medically fragile, are battling to overcome organ failure, many times needing artificial airways and ventilation, and always on the knife-edge of infection. The role of a medical speech-language pathologist in a LTACH is vastly different than in an acute care setting, far different from treating in a rehabilitation setting, and a distant planet from the speech therapist's job in the school system. For my ventilator patients, I worked closely with the respiratory therapists as well as the doctors and nurses to establish some sort of communication while the person is on a ventilator, and then after he is weaned from the vent. These patients may need ventilator maintenance for weeks: weeks of not speaking, weeks of strong sedation, weeks of not drinking or eating. These are the challenges of the LTACH SLP, who must always keep in mind how very fragile patients' bodies can be.

A speaking valve invented by an SLP can be employed during ventilator time or after weaning. My patients are deeply grateful for the ability to express themselves once more using this device. The speaking valve also minimizes air loss within the trachea, thereby maintaining the intratracheal pressure helpful in actively swallowing. I have told families that for the person with a hole in his neck, swallowing without wearing the speaking valve is like the rest of us trying to swallow with our lips open. We need that bit of pressure to push food down. Who knew?

What I surely didn't know, after working at Sumter: Could I possibly work in a hospital again? I had treated extreme residents and would now be expected to treat extreme patients. As I gathered old skills to meet the needs of this once-again new population, I drew upon my skills at videofluoroscopic swallow study and also attended coursework at a nearby university to learn how to perform fiber-optic endoscopic evaluation of swallowing. With new skills, new technology at my disposal, and years of experience, I faced a much sicker, more fragile group of patients. I have not left my neurologically impaired people behind.

The LTACH will admit some medically complex folks who start out with brain injury: they have suffered strokes or traumatic head injuries. My heart has been broken over and over treating youngsters who should be planning college, marriage, or children only to end up on ventilators with gut-wrenching bedsores and infections. When one stays long enough in a hospital room, under strong medication, burning with fever, at a loss for oxygen, one's head becomes the (hopefully) temporary home to delirium. Other patients have clouded their years with alcohol, street or prescription drugs, too much of the wrong foods and succumb to organ failure: pancreatitis, liver failure, cirrhosis, renal failure. They enter the emergency room "out of their heads" and continue in delirium as they settle into the LTACH.

Delirium is a sudden onset of disorientation, includes hallucinations, behavior fluctuation, impaired attention and short-term memory. "Sudden onset of disorientation"—reminded me of what I had experienced when I had moved to South Carolina.

Culture Shock

Little did we know that when we had traveled up I-85 into the upstate of South Carolina some eight-hundred miles in 2002, we would be leaving all that was known behind and entering a culture so different from what was familiar that it would be years before we each got our bearings. Sumter Center kept me secluded for eight to ten hours a day within those pink walls with little time to get acquainted with my new home in South Carolina. Back to work in acute care, I was again surrounded by everyday folk, neighbors in my new city who had the misfortune to get sick.

The first month on the job I saw an elderly woman in a wheelchair gesturing wildly to her mouth and then heaving a sizeable quantity of dark brown liquid all over herself and the floor. My impression was coffee-ground emesis, or violent vomiting of brown liquid that signifies organ failure. But it wasn't. Grandma just wanted a receptacle into which to spit her chewing tobacco. Down the hall, one day, I heard loud, confusing screaming. Investigating, I saw in one patient's hospital room several bib-overall-dressed people, one or two large snakes, and a woman writhing on the floor. I reported this to the nurse supervisor who, without batting an eye, informed very casually they were snake handlers.

I grew up with Eastern European immigrants. I was raised in a community of Russians, the majority (if not all) were Russian Orthodox Christians. We were bussed from our little town into Lakewood, New Jersey, which then was predominantly Jewish, and still is now. I wanted to blend in and be popular so I had to become accepted by the popular girls who were all Jewish. This was not difficult for me. Eastern Europeans (including my family) shared a great many customs, values, and food with Jewish people. What was familiar was also comfortable, and I was successful in making friends.

The same kids with whom I finished high school were the ones with whom I went to college. New York University in Greenwich Village in the '60s represented many nations. I heard much Cantonese and Arabic, saw darker-skinned classmates of the subcontinent and Africa as well as Americans from all over the country. But the girls in my dorm were mostly Jewish. My first roommate was a popular majorette from my high school; let's not be coy, these girls were the epitome of the term "Jewish-American Princess." They were spoiled, designer dressed, over-confident mature young women who believed that they owned the world. I *so* wanted to be like them.

At twenty-nine, when I had left my beloved New York for South Florida, I discovered that someone had taken the continent, stood it on its side and shook it. My first patients were a mix of backgrounds with a majority of New Yorkers. All the New Yorkers fell into South Florida. I worked in "Meeamee Bitch." The recent settlers of this beautiful unspoiled island were primarily Jewish. When I arrived, the Gold Coast above 40th Street was still a hot destination and top acts entertained at

The Fountainebleu, The Eden Roc, The Thunderbird and The Playboy Hotel. Below 40th Street was residential with two-story apartment four-plexes dotting the beachfront. The elderly rocked on front terraces getting brown as berries in the Miami sun.

The Goldsteins, Wachtels and Weintraubs of the North became the Goldsteins, Wachtels and Weintraubs of the South. I didn't have to learn my patients' culture; I knew it cold. I knew that my home health care patients would absolutely insist I eat with them. I expected without insult to be served on the non-kosher goyishe plates. I knew which subjects could be discussed and which would offend. Once when an eighty-something Jewish man asked me if I were a practicing Jew, I cut him off with: "Do you want me to treat you or pray with you?" Otherwise religion was not discussed. I knew that once I was in the door, I was to get down to business without wasting time. I was to save schmoozing for after the session. They wanted to get their therapy's worth so they timed the session then took up my time conversing later. I expected my clients to be presentable in a housedress or robe or elastic-wasted leisure pants and a top. Some would be dressed to go out, fully made up with carrot-colored teased hair, and no place to go. In sun-loving South Florida, appearance was important. Too many times I overheard: "He was just on the tennis court yesterday when my ninety-eight–year-old brother had a stroke, can you believe it?"

When I treated "old Florida colored folk," as they called themselves, I expected the men to avoid meeting my gaze, a parcel of their culture, I'm told. This made it difficult to ask them to imitate mouth postures for words, but I had to work with what they were comfortable with. In the poor black community, I was given the courtesy, needed or not, of having a child of the family "watch my car" while I was treating grandma. Medical people were prized in poor black neighborhoods. I knew that all the children in the home were not kin, but that some were taken in by neighbors to raise them as their own. I quickly learned that black and white in Florida was not the same as black and white in New York.

In the '70s, Miami Beach was just beginning to accept integration. Signs for "colored" still hung over water fountains, but were largely ignored. Private clubs still existed that did not permit blacks or women or Jews. Some dark neighborhoods did not welcome whites as I discovered very awkwardly when I entered a movie theater in Liberty City. Everyone stopped and stared at me with what I felt as hostility and not curiosity, as I entered and quickly left. My black co-workers did not know how to behave with me when I chose to sit with them at lunch rather than "my own kind."

The Mariel Boatlift of 1980 and Hurricane Andrew in 1992 had changed the playing field of South Florida in a big way. The white Jews moved North, the Blacks colonized in different neighborhoods, and the Cubans flooded Miami Dade County. I traded the Goldsteins for Gonzaleses, the Wachtels for Garcias and the Weintraubs for Vegas.

My South Carolina LTACH required one week of orientation for all new hires. One of the seminars was about Cultural Diversity. The basic message was that we were to acknowledge and be sensitive to the values, spiritual and religious beliefs, mindset, and traditions of others. I had left behind my Russian and Jewish communities long behind. I live now in a community, which is definitely Southern Baptist. I traded the Gonzaleses, the Goldsteins, the Garcias for the McKittricks, the Odums and the Snipeses. Now I say "Hey" and not "Hi." I speak softer. No I don't, who am I kidding? I try not to let my atta-control Jersey-New York mouth curse. I especially try not to say "goddamn" or "Jesus Christ." The "f" and "s" words are still acceptable in some quarters.

They speak English here, sort of. I still need translations of regionalisms and find thick dialects hard to keep up with. I now expect to be asked what church I go to when I meet someone. I still get impatient when business comes after discussion of the children, the grandchildren, the nephew's divorce, the church social, those Tigers, ailments, ailments, and ailments. I still flinch when someone yells, "Go Cocks!" Directions to places use churches as landmarks, maybe because a single street's name changes every mile or so. And streets aren't arranged in easy-to-navigate grids but twist and turn and suddenly just stop. Natives will direct one to go to where "that ole Po Mill used to be (ten years before)" leaving me with no clue what he's talking about.

We moved to a city where men walk around in bib overalls and no shirt. Where some college students dress in demur ankle-covering skirts and high necklines. After spending long years in Manhattan, with its worldwide reputation of being rude (not true) then living in South Florida where you can get shot beeping your horn (true), it was sweet to have cars stop and allow me to cross the street, to be respectfully called ma'am by everyone young or old, and to be treated gently. Southerners have wonderful manners.

When sharing life experiences with my beloved patients and their families, I have gained a strong respect for the culture of the South. Many of these folks have lived within the same town or county for generations. Southerners hold family very close, as evidenced by a family enclave of smaller houses, or more typically single-wide trailers, surrounding the original "large" house of the parents. Ask a country-born gentleman how far he has ever traveled in his life and he will probably tell you either to Myrtle Beach or Pigeon Forge. People *stay* here. Why go anywhere else?

Greenville is an amazing town with much to offer anyone. The climate is ideal with long springs and autumns although the natives will inevitably complain about the (nonexistent) humidity. South Carolinians would melt in South Florida's pea soup dampness. Serious storms normally skirt the surrounding mountains and don't threaten us with much more than a rare ice storm. Industry of all kinds continues to be relatively healthy. Homeowners joke that we must all sign a pact to go out to eat at least four times a week in order to keep the numerous restaurants going. Greenville is home to Paris Mountain and its beautiful State Park with all the amenities. A stunningly beautiful waterfall with a history of powering the once gloriously successful cotton mills runs through the center of town. A world-class theater, many smaller theatrical venues and a sports arena are nearby. But my favorite thing about Greenville is glimpsing the gray-blue Smoky Mountains like a petticoat showing through the silhouette of buildings and trees.

The sparkling, confident cities of Greenville, Spartanburg, Columbia, and Charleston ebb away and one suddenly finds oneself in deep country amidst gut-wrenching poverty, unemployment, and the loss of antebellum innocence. Rural South Carolina resembles a third-world country. My LTACH drew from these demographics as well.

Working at Sumter Center stretched my psychological and philosophical horizons. Living in the Deep South likewise exposed me to a very different way of life. Although most of my working life was spent in various hospitals, specialty or neighborhood, the hospital that now employed me was disconcertingly somehow strange.

179

There were no visiting hours; friends dropped in all the time and in numbers. Family "slept in" on window seats or recliners. It was common to see Billy-Bob's kin lying, sitting, or leaning while feeding my patient, bathing him, and gossiping with him. Sometimes families did the unexpected.

A very fragile patient, Roy G., was visited by his equally fragile, but not-hospitalized, wife. She bid him goodbye, kissed him, and left with the neighbor who drove her and the neighbor's granddaughter. We figured the group made it halfway to the interstate when the unfortunate man passed. The neighbor was reached on her cell phone and the group turned around. We saw the neighbor and her seven-year-old daughter get off the elevator, followed by Roy's widow. The charge nurse called them over to offer a coloring book or TV to the child while the adults visited the room where Roy, very dead, waited.

The widow and her neighbor declined the nurse's offer. They entered Roy's room, bringing along the neighbor's child. We wondered, *Why in heaven's name does the neighbor and her daughter want to be in the dead man's room?* We peeked. To our amazement (I told you, you can't make this stuff up!) the little girl and the widow posed seated on the bed with their arms around the head and shoulders of the now-dead Roy while the neighbor took photos. I was shocked. Then, they settled in and ate the chips and dip they had brought until the undertaker arrived. (I think the girl even offered Mr. G. a chip.)

Codependence in families was rampant. Forbidden foods were imported into patients' room. When the doctor didn't supply the amount of painkiller the patient or the spouse deemed absolutely necessary, presto. It would come from outside.

One might think that transitioning from an exotic place like Sumter to working the acute care and rehabilitation circuit might be regressing professionally, but I have been able to put my experience at Sumter to very good use. I have seen, been told of, or experienced many anomalies of medicine that the average speech pathologist or doctor has never seen. I dredge up a memory of this patient or that disorder and have a short cut to diagnosing or compiling care plans. Sumter taught me about pharmaceuticals, about psychotropics, about hypnotics, about narcotics, and the kaboom that can occur with poly-substance abuse. I have witnessed the permanent effects of drug and alcohol abuse and wish schools would take their kids on field trips to my LTACH instead of to the petting zoo.

Another patient, Mr. K, came to us with pancreatitis and an altered mental status. He had been a lifelong alcoholic. His course of recovery did not fit the expectations of his doctors. Instead of gradually waking up and shaking off his delirium, he slept constantly, was difficult to rouse, and was severely confused when he did awaken. A passing nurse caught his wife slipping something into his juice. The wife denied it but continued the practice and was again caught. A family and staff meeting was held. The wife brought her two adult children to the meeting, and the three reported that Mr. K was an ugly drunk and was physically and emotionally abusive to his family. They didn't much like him anymore. His son stated he wouldn't mind if his father did die. Mr. K was our patient, and we couldn't have sons and wives murdering our clients under our very noses.

The family was prohibited from visiting the patient. Without his wife's "loving" help, he actually recovered and was pleasant company. Administration didn't want him to return to his home, feeling he would be in danger of either returning to his evil ways, or being killed by his wife. Legally, the hospital had no choice, so Mr. K went home. He was admitted back into the emergency room within forty-eight hours, unresponsive. He ended up back in the ICU, back on a ventilator and died soon thereafter. His family either got their wish or had accomplished the intended results.

As a consequence, the LTACH became proactive. Posting a security guard outside each room wouldn't have worked, so cameras were installed in every room giving the monitor tech at the nurses' station a clear view of anything untoward going on. The camera proved a source of endless amusement for the staff. We watched, of course, bemused and horrified as a girlfriend entered her very sick honey's room and closed the door. She crawled onto his bed and they snuggled for a while. After a time, she inspected the various tubes and leads from his body to the vital signs monitors. Then, as the camera watched, she was filmed removing the man's catheter from his penis and performing fellatio to the disgust and hilarity of the staff, who couldn't bring themselves to look away from the video monitor.

Of course, not everything was captured on camera. R.W. was a lifelong smoker who had been hospitalized for lung cancer. When he graduated from his stint on the ventilator, he was able to take walks around the hall, first with the guidance of his physical therapist, and then he was given permission to stroll alone. He had an agenda. He disappeared off the floor for long-enough periods of time that no one could find him. Tobacco use of any kind is not permitted anywhere on the hospital campus so the staff wondered where R.W. had gone. Fortunately he was not as slick as our administrator, who happened to look out her window one afternoon to see R.W. relaxing under a tree right under her office window. He was given a nicotine patch, his ass-sheltering robe was confiscated, and he was forbidden to leave the floor.

Many LTACH patients languish about day after day without a soul seeing to their various legal and illegal needs. Families will either visit extensively, many times sleeping on the window seat or in the recliner, or not at all until death is imminent—then *all* the family line the halls and fill the room tripping over staff trying to tend to the still-living patients. It would have been nice if these patients would have had visits while they were alive. Veteran's families in my New York VA came once in a while, probably after therapy hours. Even before 9/11, it was difficult to gain entrance to a federal building. In Florida, visitors were respectful of posted visiting hours and did not interrupt therapy time unless asked to be present. South Carolina was different.

Different, too, was the average age of my caseload. No more ninety year olds. My southern patients' average age was in the fifties. No more suntanned wrinkled golfers or slim women in beachwear. The bulk (literally) of my southern patients was well over three hundred pounds, a medical distinction known as "super morbidly obese." Southerners joke that they fry everything. Popular restaurants are "meat and three" all-you-can-eat buffets. The LTACH had custom-made super-sized bariatric beds and chairs. The job of jockeying these folks around, or transferring them, is not a pretty one. In one case, a nurse's aide had the dubious distinction of being the one assigned to the patient's pannus: When the extra-large female patient was flopped around on her bed every two hours to prevent pressure or bed sores, this aide held and guided her drooping stomach bulk.

Still others guided breasts bigger than a pair of large sea mammals. Not only were they visually unappealing, our overweight patients had not been able to perform basic hygiene very effectively for years. The skin in the deep folds of their flesh had begun to rot. In one man's crotch, a nurse found the TV remote he had misplaced days earlier at his home.

Charts were rubber-stamped (or should have been) with the ubiquitous legend, "Super morbidly obese, diabetes, end stage renal failure, respiratory failure." I asked my own doctor very seriously when I could expect end-stage renal failure to begin. She assured me some people actually make it to old age without their kidneys pooping out on them.

∽

George was supposed to go home that afternoon. He still had been receiving a specialized diet and the doctor asked me to evaluate whether that diet could be changed. George was sitting up in bed, already dressed in street clothes, watching TV, impatient to be picked up. I turned his TV off, re-introduced myself and placed my clipboard down on his bed. I turned on my penlight, and asked him to open his mouth. And I saw what looked for all the world like a mouse running up a wall under the wallpaper, *in his mouth! Curious,* I thought.

I turned to note this on my clipboard when the patient made a "kkkrch!" sound. In the instant I turned back to him, his color changed and I realized he was dying. I yelled for help, "Code Blue!" I primed myself for a harrowing session of rigorous CPR. The nurse took quick vitals and pronounced him. I then realized with an icy feeling that I had witnessed a stroke. The "mouse" running up the wall of his mouth was a thrombus in his carotid artery.

Witnessing a stroke while it happens was not a welcome way of enhancing my professional resume. But I padded my work experience in other exotic ways. I listened, paid attention, and stored nuggets of exotica away. I remember a fifty-year-old woman in a Florida hospital who was referred to me after she suddenly lost both her voice and her ability to swallow. The subsequent workup by her doctor revealed an aggressive adenocarcinoma in the upper lobe of her left lung. I wondered about the connection. I had known from my neurology and anatomy courses that the cranial nerves provided muscle power and sensation to the areas of the mouth and throat I worked with every day. I traced the tenth cranial nerve away from the larynx and discovered it indeed meandered through the top of the left lung with connections that influenced breathing and the way the heart works. I asked a radiologist to "tour" me through my patient's chest X-ray. He pointed out that the lung cancer had surrounded a portion of this woman's tenth cranial nerve, effectively cutting off enervation to her larynx.

Twenty years later, another patient of mine arrived to the hospital with a sudden loss of voice and swallowing. I told my doctor to do a CT of the lungs. He found the cancer. He looked at me curiously: "How did you know?"

Bingo, I thought. *I'm a genius.*

I *love* working in hospitals. I love the sounds: the urgency of a ventilation monitor; the wheedle-wheedle of phones; the insistence of ding-ding-ding of IV pumps when they're empty; the high pitched beep-beep requesting help, patient's groans, the suck-suck splash noise of someone's trach being suctioned; the murmur of visitors in rooms; the odd clack-clack of heels since we all wear rubber soles; the raucous laughter of the staff warding away thoughts of the seriousness of their work; and the overhead voice alerts summoning all who are near to hurry to a cardiac arrest, or immediate stroke, or a suspected fire.

I don't so much love the smells. Basically, there are no smells because hospitals are sanitized, and then there's the odor of feces, but not for long since feces is cleaned up right away. Up close, people who have lain in beds awhile stink. Infections really stink, some unbearably. Personnel might have a dab of cologne on and that breaks up the no-smell stretch. I don't like the smell or feel of the disinfectant gel that hangs in every room and we can't go in or out of any room without disinfecting our hands *all the time*. The stuff I use to sterilize my FEES endoscope smells strongly like bleach. But the day is mostly smell-less.

I like the urgency of a health crisis which is not my own. Hospitals have many areas where outsiders are not allowed. I like that people with things to fix get fixed. I like wearing pajamas (scrubs) to work. Today, I still get excited when we admit an individual with a diagnosis of stroke or closed head injury; I can diagnose and treat these folks blindfolded. The fact that my neurology patients are further compromised by comorbidities means I need to step up my game and not become complacent.

Complex comorbidities scare the crap out of me. As is appropriate, when one is young, the frailties of illness or age or both are beyond our horizons. Middle age teaches us the earth is indeed round. The horizon is not as distant as we once hoped. At the LTACH, the nurses and therapists interrupt documentation or calls from families or

medication justification to muse: "How would *we* do it?"
What are the limits of our resources? What is the depth of pain
we choose to endure? The "we" then becomes "I" in the early morning
before I hear the alarm clock, or in the quiet walks around a lake alone,
or lovingly beholding the peace of a sleeping child. I told myself I
needed to consider my options. Just. In. Case. The discussion of my
options is acceptable to my spouse as he considers his own and ours. The
discussion of my options drives my young son crazy. A palmist told my
mother when she was in her sixties that she would die at seventy-two
years of age. Her brothers died at seventy-two (no, they didn't but this is
her superstition.) On her seventieth birthday, she began to gather the
dress and jewelry in which she would be buried. Every couple of months
she would insist that I accompany her to the chosen funeral home to pick
out a suitable casket. At first, appalled and saddened, I teared up and
shooed her morbid plan away. After several fruitless trips to that funeral
home, I saw the humor in the idea that one could calendar one's own
natural death. Trips to the funeral home had become blackly comic, a
reason to tease. On my mother's seventy-fifth birthday when she was
flirting, or already in bed with madness, I really didn't know if she
realized she made it past her seventy-second year and was still on this
earth—or on her own planet of dementia.

"Draw a line. This is your life. Now mark on it where you are
now." My therapist-friend, Natalie's horizontal lifeline teases me with its
possibilities. But it is only a lifeline. It can't predict the terrain I will
journey through until my end. My patients have taught me how tensile-
steel resilient humans can be. My patients have taught me how to justify
being alive when everything argues against life. My work has educated
me. In my sixties, I know about complex comorbidities, how the elegant
design of our anatomies can tip one way or the other. How fight-or-flight
can become an insidious destruction of one organ after another, allowing
infection to pillage.

Whether or not any of us plan to be struck down in one fashion
or another, we need to anticipate the contingencies. *When is being alive
no longer our choice? Who gets to decide if we no longer have the
consciousness or the wherewithal to make important medical decisions?
How many organs can we abide losing? Is there any hope? Can I get
better? Is better all it is cracked up to be? Is 'hope' all it's cracked up to
be?* Surviving can be a lonely, monotonous, unproductive place. Or not.

Survivors receive no headlines, no monuments, no knowledge of what they went through to survive, to continue to live. The dead are everlasting. We carve their names on granite and mark their deaths in raised-bronze letters. We mourn, celebrate, extol, and write headlines to mark the passing of those who have passed. The dead are given *names*. "A bus hit a sedan on Highway 101 last night. The *injured* were taken to the local hospital. Their condition is deemed serious." No names. What about the "merely" injured? With few exceptions, survivors are quickly forgotten. They have no monuments. The broken stagger, crawl, or are shipped back from war, from horrific car accidents, from street fights, near-drownings, from strokes.

Some survivors are fortunate. The wounded live on and are cherished by loved ones, pitied by strangers, and cared for by doctors, nurses, therapists, and assorted other beleaguered caregivers. Do we track the progress of the broken? James Brady and Gabby Gifford provide exceptions. We watched the gunshots that brought them down. Through the magic of the media we see them again later, alive, eyes open, standing, speaking; but what did it take to get these two respected public servants back? Patricia Neal, Dick Clark, and Kirk Douglas. These are brave souls who didn't let a stroke destroy the days allotted to them, but plowed on in the public eye. What challenges did they overcome in their struggle to return home? A neurological event is a game changer.

My approach hasn't changed that much through the years although the seriousness of the LTACH person's condition has. Upon receiving an order to treat, I ferret out every bit of information I can gather about my patient. If the patient does not come to us with a packet of information—discharge summary, progress notes, drug list, evaluations from therapists, pertinent medical history—I look up the next of kin specified and call them to get information, I look them up on the computer, or I seek out the doctor attending. Only then do I make my approach.

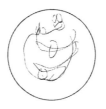

NOVEMBER, 2005

LTACH ROOM 1012

Shirley

I entered the room. The woman wasn't moving. She was lying on her side with a foam wedge beneath her to support her. She was turned every two hours to prevent her bedsores from getting worse. I told her that I was raising the bed up. I raised the entire bed to a height comfortable for me to see her face-to-face so that I didn't have to bend. I told her: "My name is Lydia, what is yours?" She didn't answer me. I touched her arm and her cheek.

"Is your name Shirley?" No response. I said, "Your name is Shirley, mine is Lydia. Could you open your eyes?" She opened her eyes. They didn't look at me but stared into the space behind me.

I said, "Can you find my face?" When the woman looked into my eyes I walked slowly around the bed. She didn't follow me with her eyes. I came back to her side.

I asked, "Do you know where you are?"

She very subtly furrowed her brow.

I told her, "You are in the hospital. You are in Greenville, which is in South Carolina. Where do you live? Do you live in Greenville?"

I got no response.

I go on. "This is a hospital in Greenville, South Carolina. It is 2005. This month is November."

The woman didn't respond. She closed her eyes. I ask her to stay awake and to find my face. She didn't respond. Shirley's stroke involved a respiratory arrest. I now added lack of oxygen for an undetermined amount of time to the cause of damage done by the bleed. This was a

187

new brand of stroke for me—deeper, more involved, requiring my infinite patience. I had trouble channeling Bea, Nat's mom Doris, Leonard, or the thousands of past stroke victims. I filled a sterile glove with the ice I had brought in. I tied the thumb together with the wrist to make an icepack. I stroked Shirley's cheek with the ice. She opened her eyes.

I told her to find my face and I say, "My name is Lydia, tell me your name." This may be the only thing I would get this session. I wrote my note for the visit saying "patient rouses to sound, opens eyes, and makes brief eye contact." She did not visually track, and her attention span was short. She provided no attempt to speak and she didn't follow commands other than to find my face. I told the doctor in my note that she seemed to be a Rancho Los Amigos Level II. Like the Glascow Coma Scale, the Rancho was a scale of five descriptions of the levels of consciousness. It is used primarily for closed head injuries resulting in a coma. In this case, I was using it to describe the performance of a patient who had sustained massive bleeding in the brain resulting in cardiac and respiratory arrest with hypoxia.

Even after treating hundreds of patients in similar dire circumstances, I can't say with certainty how much of Shirley would return. It's a crap shoot. There were too many variables: death of brain cells that have drowned in the original bleeding; loss of brain cells due to lack of oxygen for an unknown period of time while patient suffered cardiac and respiratory arrest; what the patient was like before the events devastated her; whether or not the body's responses to catastrophe have persisted , now working against getting better, sapping strength and other resources; whether this patient's immune system can rally or whether she loses function of other vital organs such as her kidneys and liver. My role was to keep on treating this patient savoring every tiny response she made to me.

Day two with Shirley was the same as day one. On day three, Shirley's eyes found my face and stayed with me as I walked away from her. I thought I saw a mere hint of a smile. Her fingers flicked ever-so-slightly despite that she remained a functional quadriplegic and all four limbs were so weak she couldn't move them; this was not due to spinal cord injury but due to the debility caused by organ failure and sustained suffering.

I asked for her hand. I picked up her hand and asked her to

squeeze mine. Did she? I couldn't tell. Because Shirley was maintaining her gaze at my face, I decided her attention was good enough for me to siphon a drop or two of water into a straw and place it just inside her lips. She purses her lips and clamps her teeth but the water entered her mouth and she swallowed after a while. I asked her if she liked the water. She nodded. I asked her to open her lips for more water. She did not respond. I again siphoned water with a straw and that time she didn't clamp her teeth. She swallowed. I asked her if she wanted more.

"Say 'more', Shirley, 'more, more'."

She continued to gaze at me but didn't make an attempt to speak. I asked her to open her lips and modeled this for her with my face. Shirley is a large, "morbidly obese" African-American woman in her early fifties who had no teeth or dentures. She now had a habit of pulling her lips into her mouth with the result that they were hopelessly chapped and coated with old, congealed lip balm. She stared at me and unlocked the pressure on her lips but they didn't open all the way; I got just a peek and then she went back to folding them into the safety of her mouth.

I asked, "Can you open your mouth like this 'ahhhh'," and she gave a slight smile and shrugged. It was progress; I got a meaningful though vague response to a command. And my mother said I had no patience.

On day ten, "Hi, Miss Shirley," got me a smile and a direct gaze. I looked her over. This time she was positioned leaning toward the door with wedges and pillows so she could see who came into her room.

I comment, "Your nails are getting long, you need a manicure." She raised one hand limply to peer at it and gave me one of her signature shrugs. I promised her I would bring my stuff and do her nails tomorrow. I asked if she wanted red or pink. She mouths "pink."

Shirley came to us with her breathing still supported by a ventilator. She had a tracheostomy tube in her throat but by then it had a clear-colored cap or cover on it. I knew that she was now using her nose and mouth to breathe and had the possibility of using her voice. We had not been successful in getting vocalized speech only her coughs are audible. I didn't want to give her any more than a tiny ice chip or a couple cc's of water since no voice might mean her vocal cords do not come together and if they do not come together, sitting atop her airway as they were, they weren't likely to protect her airway. I noticed that the little bit she got from me by mouth is quickly swallowed. It was a good sign.

LTACH Room 1014: Tawana

Next door to Shirley was Tawana, a forty-year-old kindergarten teacher who collapsed on the playground one day. At her age, she could have been friends with Rosa, Ashley, or Debbie, the young women I treated in the '80s. She was brought to the hospital and diagnosed with brain hemorrhage. She stayed in a coma for three days and was, like Shirley, placed on a ventilator. She greeted folks who entered her room with a direct challenging stare. She was constantly in motion trying to remove tubes, lines, IVs, and trachs, an activity that earned her wrist restraints since the nurses really don't like replacing difficult to insert tubes and other items. Whatever was said to her resulted in a nod, for all the world as if she were agreeing or at least understood. Her family was convinced she "conversed" with them and Tawana had at least one nurse who felt she was depressed and "spiteful." I loved that one.

One look at her brain scan results told me she had bilateral subcortex and two lobes of her right hemisphere necrosed from the bleed. This constituted much of her brain's association cortex or, in layman's terms, the logistics center, the highway system, which connects town to town.

Upon helping Tawana eat one day, her mom said, "I bet it's hard to get used to eating with her right hand. She's left-handed." This statement made me think: I recalled a neurology seminar I had attended years before where it was postulated that if a left-handed person wrote with the wrist bent and the hand cocked, he or she was left brain dominant—like a great majority of the population. However, if the left-handed writer wrote with no bend to the wrist, this indicated that the dominance was in the right brain since, I had always supposed, the dominant side controlling the act of symbolic graphics connected more efficiently with the contralateral, or opposite, side. This got me thinking.

I decided to complete a strict formal evaluation of Tawana's residual communication and language skills from the very basic level through more complex, over-learned material to combination stimuli (gesture + speech, written word + object, etc.), I considered three dynamics: a) Tawana is basically uncooperative with formal testing; b) Tawana is more impaired than she lets on; c) I wasn't using the right kind of evaluation tools. I went with "c."

I elected to merely inhabit the room with Tawana and observe her actions carefully without insinuating myself. She showed much of her premorbid personality: she glanced in the mirror and primped her hair, she glanced at me to see what I was doing, she continued to evade her restraints despite that they were no longer on her, she pointed to her bed indicating that she wanted to lie down again, and she reacted to people passing in the hall by craning to see who they were. Yet when I asked her to do something, she merely nodded. I took my informal observation to mealtime. I figured most of us were motivated by hunger, and if hungry, we would use tried-and-true means to accomplish eating. When I placed Tawana's tray in front of her, she clearly wanted to eat, yet she sat there and looked at all the stuff on her tray without touching anything.

I verbally instructed her to pick up her fork. I took care not to look at the fork or gesture to it, or hand it to her. She nodded. She did not go for the fork. I opened my mouth wide and pointed to the food, a clear signal I wanted her to eat. She nodded. I speared some food onto her fork and held it to her mouth. She turned away and pursed her lips. I put the fork closer to her nose and pantomimed smelling. She did. Then she opened her mouth for the fork. I delivered the fork to her mouth and left it there. After a beat or two sitting with the fork dangling out of her mouth, Tawana reached for the fork.

She held it as she used to, in the correct position. I pantomimed spearing up more food. She stared at my face and even bent towards me. To hear? To see what I was saying? I decided upon, "to try to understand my words." After a few more forkfuls of food left dangling in her mouth, she began to remove the fork from her lips and spear more food, eventually bringing the food to her mouth. I gathered much information about Tawana in that one mealtime. I learned that she could initiate a request (pointing to her bed for me to help her lie down). I learned that her stares served a purpose of trying to understand what was said to her. I also learned that she lost the ability to make her body move to accomplish the most familiar tasks like eating.

Several more sit-and-watch sessions told me that Tawana took regular "time-outs" in which her attention would lapse and she would either sit and do nothing or repeat what she had already done. A good example was the time I handed Tawana a toothbrush. She did not hold it the old way she once did, but gripped it somehow and put it in her mouth, rubbing her teeth with the plastic side. When she was finished "brushing" her teeth, I handed her a small hand-held mirror. She proceeded to brush her teeth with the mirror. I handed her a spoon and she brushed her teeth with the spoon.

Putting all these clues together, I now put a long-ago learned label on Tawana's behavior: she presented a global aphasia, in which both understanding and expressing skills are impacted; emerging into a mainly receptive aphasia, which she expressed through meaningful gestures and eventually words but had more difficulty figuring out what others said to her; combined with a dense (serious) verbal and ideational apraxia, which meant figuring out how to go from intention to action using, respectively, spoken expression and manipulating familiar objects correctly.

Our LTACH had a portion of one floor decorated like a slice of Main Street with an outdoor produce stand next to a grocery window next to a bank with a teller's window. I had been struggling with a dignified-looking gentleman who came to the LTACH after he had suffered a stroke. His body did not seem to be affected: no arm hung limp and he could walk with minimal assistance. This gentleman was always with his doting wife who would help him out of his bed and into the chair in his room. There he would sit zombie-like, unmoving, and staring ahead. He flicked little glances at me but would not engage.

Going through my repertoire, I provided commands, open-ended sentences meant to elicit his name and hometown and I named relative items: "nose," "shirt," "pen," etc. Nothing. I walked over to the mock Main Street and gathered up three pieces of plastic fruit. I held up a banana: "Banana, I eat a—" Nothing. "Apple, take a bite of—"

Nothing. The wife was beginning to shift in her seat looking uncomfortable.

Leaning on what I thought would be automatic, I said, "Catch!" while tossing him the apple.

He made no attempt to catch it or deflect it.

To my embarrassment, the apple bonked my patient on the head as he sat there unmoving. The wife began to quietly cry. The next day, some of my co-workers teased me, saying I did therapy by throwing fruit at my patients. Sometimes the magic worked, and sometimes it didn't.

A medical truth is that if you have seen one stroke, you've only seen one stroke. Given the character of the stroke, the part of the brain affected, the extent of the lesion, the person's education, personality, age, etc., each stroke is different. One person's stroke can't be compared with another's. Similarly, one gunshot wound to the head is very different than another's for some of the same reasons, and for other reasons. Treating and being dramatically impacted by knowing Sheila did not prepare me for treating Rayshun.

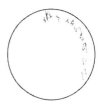

FEBRUARY, 2010

LTACH ROOM 1020

Ray

Charles Rayshun Sullivan , or Ray as his friends knew him, was in the wrong place at the wrong time. A senior, looking forward to graduating in December from Tusculum College with a degree in sports management, Ray decided to visit his parents while waiting for his new apartment to become vacant. His mother, Carolyn, tried to dissuade him from coming home: "I knew something bad was gonna' happen," she had said. While home for that weekend in July, Ray was asked to pick up his cousin at a club in town. He was caught in the crossfire of a gang dispute.

Carolyn was asleep. She woke suddenly feeling cool air brush her face. She arose to check on the household. Her daughter, Sheena, had answered the phone call from the hospital. She erupted out of her room and had begun banging on Carolyn's door.

"Ray's been shot in the face!" she screamed.

When the family arrived at the hospital, Ray was still alert. He was lying on a gurney with his head bandaged. He thrashed his head back against the gurney again and again, "Mom it hurts so bad!" Blood soaked the bandage and poured into Ray's eyes. The emergency room physician stopped by to tell the Sullivans, "We just got another gunshot victim in. We're going to take him into surgery first, then your son."

The other victim was Ray's shooter, the gang leader. The hospital personnel assumed they were dealing with two gang members. Mute, helpless rage combined with worry and concern about Ray's future—were they really going to keep Ray waiting while they saved the life of his shooter?

After his surgery, Ray stayed in the hospital for two months tethered to monitors and IV pumps, and to a ventilator by an endotracheal tube. His mother, Carolyn, can recall pushing him around the medical floor in a wheelchair when Ray suddenly had a seizure. Because of that event, she chose to stay with her son. Her boss fired her for missing too much work. "What was I supposed to do? Ray needed me."

When he was stable, Ray was transferred to my LTACH. The floor staff was abuzz with the expectation of dealing with a gunshot victim so young. We never really got the chance: Ray was transferred out in two days to have yet another procedure to remove a mass in his sinus cavity. He went from that hospital directly to a rehabilitation center in Atlanta.

On Thanksgiving Day, a day for giving thanks in so many ways, Ray was brought back to his home via ambulance from Atlanta. In newspaper photos he resembled a concentration camp victim lying on the gurney in his parents' front lawn. His parents, Carolyn and Charles were beyond ecstatic. Both put their own lives aside to strengthen and nurture Ray. His father, Charles, supported Ray as he walked around the house and yard holding onto a walker. At this time, Ray was able to converse in bursts of one to three words. He shared Thanksgiving dinner with his family and was starting to gain his strength back while working to gain back his weight.

On Christmas Eve of 2009, Carolyn reported that Ray was listless and sweaty, "moping on the couch." He had a temperature of 104 degrees. His doctor in Atlanta insisted they bypass the local ER and bring him back to Atlanta as fast as possible. The staff was waiting and ready for Ray. Carolyn and Charles left for the night, assured that Ray was going to get better.

A bright-colored Contact Precaution sign on Ray's closed door greeted them the next morning. The staff was dressed in personal protection garb and looked like aliens. Carolyn was mystified and angry that no one from the hospital had called to tell them how grave Ray's situation was. A pump, which had been inserted into Ray's side to insure a steady flow of baclofen (a muscle relaxer used to treat muscle symptoms including spasm, pain, and stiffness) had become infected with what the public has come to know as "MRSA", or methicillin-resistant Staphylococcus aureus. MRSA is a "staph" germ that doesn't improve with the typical first-line antibiotics that usually cure staph infections. The infection and removal of much-needed baclofen caused Ray to "shut down," according to Carolyn. "He stopped speaking. He couldn't move. His body became stiff. He was unable to eat. He was losing valuable weight despite that he was receiving liquid food through the tube in his belly. I called his doctors and they just said blend some 'real' food and put that in his feeding tube. We were trying to put some weight on him." When Ray was again medically stable but not ready yet to go home, he returned to our LTACH.

In February 2010, I recall my twenty-three-year-old patient as emaciated with stick-like arms bent upward on his chest. His mother and father took turns staying with him. Each eagerly invited tips on what they could do to help their only son. Ray's parents impressed everyone with their tireless efforts at helping Ray. His dad worked his limbs constantly, rubbing and teasing each arm or leg away from the position the stiffness imprisoned. While the hospital's therapists were limited by ethics and "good practice" treatment, my patient's family crossed boundaries in how they handled Ray. Whatever the physical therapists taught, Ray's parents followed through on—and then went much further.

I stood and watched with his physical therapist as Charles struggled to lift Ray's board-like body out of his bed. Dad forcibly bent Ray to fit him into a wheelchair despite that bending into a seated position was out of the question. We were not going to take the chance of breaking bones. With the same kind of dogged independence and persistence of my long-ago patient Anna, Ray's father developed his own brand of therapy tempered by an unequalled love for his son. When I had treated Sheila, I was childless. When I met Ray and his parents, I had a son of my own. How far would I go to bring my own Ian back to health? Was I made of the same optimistic persistence of Ray's mom? How did she hold her own life together while totally embracing her son's recovery? With all that I have seen, was I built of the same dogged optimism? I've never been so tested, I am grateful to say.

Ray's mother had had her own trials to contend with. She was convinced that had she not succeeded with her own journey, she would not have had the spiritual strength to care for Ray. A year and some months before Ray's gunshot, Carolyn left work with a backache. She went to the urgent care center to get checked out and found she had shingles, her left breast was lumpy, and her right nipple oozed pus. She left the center with an appointment for a workup at the hospital later that week. That workup revealed advanced cancer in both breasts. Scared to miss work and to schedule much-needed immediate surgery, Carolyn delayed. That first night she dreamed she was at the hospital coming out of the operating suite with her eyes open and pain free. She knew then she would be all right. Carolyn has been cancer free since 2008.

In my LTACH, Ray remained shut down. My treatment was limited. Ray turned his eyes when I entered his room and called his name. He followed my movement around his bed, but then lost interest and stared ahead. He blinked when I asked him to. He opened his mouth a couple of the times I asked. He tried to stick out his tongue for me. I tried everything in my bag of tricks to stimulate any residual communication he had in him.

I mystified his parents by assigning Ray blow-toys to reacquaint him with his mouth again. Carolyn confessed later that she thought I was a little crazy: "What did she think Ray would do with those silly horns?" I had him lick popsicles and move a lollipop with his tongue from one cheek to the other. His parents asked that I evaluate his ability to eat. Apparently, by the time Ray left rehab in Atlanta, he could take a couple supported steps and had been on a diet of solid food. When I performed an endoscopy on Ray, I noted that he swallowed some of the time, but apparently lost his fragile attention and shut down other times, allowing food to remain in his mouth or partway down his throat which was not a safe situation. I had hoped that stimulation of his attention would enable Ray to stay involved and be safe to eat. Ray left after a month and again went home. I stayed in touch with him through his home health speech pathologist.

That fall, I was paged to come to the front desk to see a visitor. A gentleman and a woman pushed a well-nourished, poised man in a wheelchair toward me. I didn't recognize the man seated in the wheelchair, but I knew the man pushing him and gasped. I knew Ray's mom and dad so the young man in the chair had to be Ray. But no, how could it be? This man was of normal weight, looked very hale and strong. He sat easily, casually, in the chair—and smiled up at me. He took out a greeting card and read aloud to the staff gathered around who had cared for him. He thanked us for all we had done for him. I don't know the exact words; I was lost in amazement and awe. I was crying tears of joy. Miracles really do happen.

I love the families of my patients. Most of the time families really care. They listen carefully to my education sessions and help the patient do the language or swallowing exercises I leave. I take great care explaining who I am and what role I play in their loved one's recovery. I joke that I am their new best friend. And I am when I give them their first piece of ice or drink of water when they have come off the ventilator. I am when I apply a speaking valve on their tracheostomy tube and they hear their own voice for the first time since returning to consciousness.

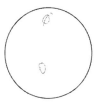

LTACH ROOM 1032

Audrey

I keep another patient and family close to my heart. Her perfect teeth were too big for her tiny face. Her eyes were closed and wouldn't open for many days. She lay curled into a fetal position, reminding me of my coma patient, Shelly, so long ago. The bed coverings outlined the sharp contours of her hip joints. Later, her family and many friends would Scotch tape photographs of her before her car accident on the walls surrounding her bed. The contrast between the vibrant, pretty redhead and the malnourished sad figure in the bed was disturbing. She was twenty-two. I stared at her for a while, and then said, "Hi Audrey, my name is Lydia. I'm your new speech therapist."

After the emergency room, Audrey was admitted to hospital, and then went to rehabilitation, then went home, was readmitted to emergency room, and now six months after her accident, on the eve of her twenty-second birthday, was admitted to my LTACH.

My evaluation and early attempts at coma stimulation were frequently interrupted by her high fevers and constant diarrhea, which compromised her fragile digestive system. She lay every once in a while twitching. The twitching developed into thrashing as Audrey shed her fevers and grew stronger. Eventually the staff needed to pack her into bed with side bolsters and pillows to help position her off her bottom so her bedsores would heal, and to prevent her from kicking her way off the side of the bed. When Audrey finally succeeded in dislodging the cumbersome, large bolster and flinging it with her good leg across the room—as a source of her own amusement, I'm sure—I figured it was time to ramp up my involvement with her.

On Day 23, her eyes were now open, sky blue and expressionless, and too large for her face. She was all teeth and blue

199

eyes. Those eyes found me at the side of her bed and followed me as I circled. When I came too close to her face she shut her eyes, shutting me out of her world.

I watched her with her visitors. She had a lot of visitors. Over the month, Audrey's room gathered more and more items—bath soaps, shampoos, lots of stuffed animals, a plush zebra-print bed covering, more photos, many cards, and some balloons. It was definitely the room of a young twenty-something girly-girl.

I requested and received her specially outfitted wheelchair from her parents who drove it from her rehabilitation hospital in Atlanta where it was left. With the group effort of Audrey's nurses, my favorite physical therapy assistant, and Audrey's occupational therapy assistant, we got her dressed and ensconced in her wheelchair. I took her for rides around the hospital. One favorite destination for the two of us was the serenity garden with its gentle waterfalls. Here I would sit on a bench close to Audrey in her wheelchair and converse with her. I babbled on, occasionally asking her for a response. She watched me and moved her mouth. Was it an attempt to speak? With her speaking valve on her trach, she had a vocalized cough and once or twice I heard her involuntarily sigh. I instructed her to cough. No success. I ratcheted it down a bit, I asked her to purr. I demonstrated purring, a slight noise in the throat, a little throat-clear number. She watched me. Later, I passed her room and stopped to say hello to her father who was sitting at her bedside. Audrey was curled in her usual fetal position and her big blue eyes looked up at me. I swear I saw the hint of a flirty smile before she took a full breath and...purred. "Dad," I said, "she did that for you."

We continued to work on talking but each speech attempt resulted in a whole-body energy burst that left Audrey exhausted. It was around this time I saw Audrey sign "I love you" to her boyfriend. I got out my trusty white board and gave Audrey the thick marker in her good right hand. She dropped it. I wrote "Greenville" and "Texas" on the white board and asked her to tell me where she was. Her tapered fingers trembled their way over to the "Greenville." Next I wrote "March" "October" and she identified the correct month. I wrote a short instruction, "Show me one finger." She did. I later broke the news to her folks that she could read and was fully oriented.

Over time Audrey developed enough strength to use her blow toys and to follow commands involving her mouth. I asked her if she was ready for an ice chip, and panic took over; she shook her head and went into a whole-body spasm. I pushed a tiny ice chip between her lips. She pushed it out. I found another small ice chip and put it in her mouth. She spit it out. I rubbed a flavored ice pop on her lips. She licked her lips. Several days later I again brought ice chips. I pushed one in her lips. She accepted the fourth one and moved it around in her mouth for a while. I noted an acceptable swallow. I gave her another crack at an ice pop. I wrapped the wooden stick in a wad of washcloth and put it in her hand. I lifted her hand to her face. She jutted her chin forward and stuck out her tongue. We got through half a cherry-flavored popsicle that day.

After many sessions, I deemed Audrey ready for endoscopy to test her swallowing skills. She tolerated small presentations of pudding and managed spooned water. I continued to combine holding foods in her hand and helping her bring food to her mouth: a primitive but effective human habit. Her pre-feeding treatments as well as her emerging eating in turn strengthened her speech. Audrey delighted in taking a deep breath and saying a high-pitched airy "Hi!" to each nurse she recognized (all of them) as I wheeled her around the hospital halls. I knew the better she got, the quicker I would lose her. The rehab center in Atlanta, where Audrey had success several long months ago gave us a goal of getting her to at least a Rancho Los Amigos Level IV. She was a solid IV and was to be visited by the rehab center's liaison the next week.

Not a day went by that we wondered about Audrey and how she was doing. I felt I had a stake, an investment, in her future. Left to our imaginations we painted her days full of frisking zebras with light blue big eyes. We pictured her coming back to see us all detailed up, nails polished smelling like her vanilla scented shampoo, and walking. She would be walking. God we loved it when our success stories came back.

Christmas brought us Shirley. Her family wheeled her in and she proudly got out of her wheelchair and hugged us all. She had new dentures and didn't suck in her lips, which were chapped no longer but a pretty rose color. Christmas brought us a card and pictures from Warren—a show-stopping before-and-after of Warren in the hospital bed tethered to his vent and IVs, next to Warren smiling from his tree-shaded back yard. But where was Audrey?

Audrey was re-admitted to our LTACH just before spring. She made it home after rehab, and then developed an infection. Our Audrey had lost more weight from her already-scant frame. She was responsive but she no longer opened her eyes. Where were all the gifts she gave us? The purring, the licking of popsicles, the serenity in the garden just the two of us, the hope. I would have to start all over again, maybe not from scratch, with the girl who arrived in light coma, non-interactive, lying in fetal position, unaware. I would go slow, of course. I would be patient.

Audrey needed to get stronger and she needed to gain some weight. I had a little more than one week before her twenty-third birthday. My gift to her was the promise of enjoying ice cream and birthday cake. I got her there before. She had been able to eat some. She could once upon a time speak in her whispery voice, and tell us how it was to be her.

We would do it again, girlfriend, I thought. *Just help me help you.*

The constant shaking and jerking used up every calorie her body took in through her feeding tube and IVs. Her gastrointestinal organs seemed to go first: the endless vicious diarrhea wasting the precious water her kidneys needed. We worked again with the whiteboard. I wrote down choices and asked her pick one. She struggled to lift her hand to the words I wrote. I struggled along with her to find an easier way for her to communicate. I had to get her there. I had to.

Audrey's nurses started a count-down poster: five days until your birthday. We noted four days, then three, then two. Her sisters pounced on her room putting up zebra birthday decorations and flowers and photos and lots of pink. Audrey's birthday was on a Friday and she was dressed and put in her wheelchair. Her mom and sister were with her. Her guests would arrive after their jobs and the celebration of Audrey would begin. But I left work for the day, and for the week.

Monday morning the decorations were still up in her room. Audrey was in her bed and the news was not good. She had vomited her tube feeding and breathed some in. She had pneumonia once more along with a gut that would not absorb the nourishment she was given. She was taken down to the radiology department for some tests. Her father went with her alongside her gurney. They were gone but a moment when her respiratory therapist was paged down "stat." I went along. Audrey had some effortful breathing but her numbers looked good, so we tended to her and left her to come back upstairs. We heard the announcement overhead "Code Blue Radiology Room 3" (the code for an arrest). Audrey had crashed and needed CPR. The whole hospital held a collective breath. An eternity later, her parents glumly got off the elevator, "They're bringing her back up."

Little girl, birthday girl, lay still, stiller than she ever did before, no twitching, no jerking, eyes closed, letting the ventilator next to her bed do the breathing for her. Whispered conversations of the nurses and therapists filled the hours, "Why won't her parents let her go?" "She won't make it this time." "Can't her family see how sick she is?" I thought of Shelly laying in her family room, her mother celebrating every twitch. I relived how harshly I had judged her parents. Now I am a parent. Could I let my child die? Should I allow my child to die? My inner debate was stupid. I fought for Audrey to make it. She was not my blood child and yet I fought for her anyway. What decision could I make if it was I sitting at the bedside of my child, holding his hand?

I passed Audrey's room and visited with her and her family and boyfriend as they prayed. "She's strong, Audrey is," her mother pleaded. I knew differently. I walked away from her room and heard a high-pitched keening behind me that didn't seem to end. I knew that voice, but also knew that it couldn't be. The voice didn't belong to Audrey anymore. I went to her bedside and she lay keening, unable to find peace, unable to find comfort in obvious pain. *What to do? What can I do?* I wondered.

I think her keening was "goodbye."

Sometimes my patients return to say "hi," to say "thank you." Sometimes they return to brag and show off their good fortune recovering.

Sometimes they don't.

Like stamps in a passport, or photos of places been, patients leave pieces of themselves in my heart. I, too, have come a long way. I am a seasoned, experienced professional with far more confidence than I had had in my early days. I will never know if I chose the right profession—it hasn't always felt like a good fit. But I know that the last several decades have been rich for me because of the people I've touched. I could have been a lighting designer on Broadway, or a full-time writer, or a record company executive—and look what I would have missed.

Friends. I know this. I know without a doubt that I have touched people—they've told me so in many, many ways. It was *mutual*.

Introductions became building rapport, became effective treatment, became stronger rapport, became love and friendship and back to health for my new friend. I continue to follow my colleague Ellen's advice. I treat every patient, every client as my own child. One crusty, outspoken old man told me, "I like you because you give a damn." So, Lydia (I have to keep telling myself), despite the burnouts, despite the crummy bosses, despite corporate politics and back-stabbing colleagues, maybe— just maybe—it's a good thing you've chosen to treat people.

I visited my gunshot victim, Ray, recently at his parents' home here in South Carolina. Photographs of the two children he fathered before his shooting set on the TV.

"They live with their mom. I can't take care of them. Do I see them as much as I want? Ahhh, no...I guess not."

Carolyn remains out of work, and stays home to care for Ray.

"I need to be able to walk without someone holding me," Ray says, and then adds confidently, "Then I plan on going back to school. I have three credits to make up then I graduate with a degree in sports management. I want to be a football coach."

When I asked what he did to pass the time, Ray said, "I exercise, I watch TV," and he continued as he laughed, "I eat. I gained too much weight trying to get back the weight I lost."

I asked what had happened to the friends that crowded the hospital waiting room the days after the shooting.

"Nah, they don't come 'round. No one visits anymore."

As I was saying my goodbyes, Ray asked his mother to bring him his favorite snack. He glimmered up at me from his armchair, "I still love my popsicles."

AFTERWORD

S peech-language pathologists attempt to provide hope and comfort by proving that broken brains can be mended. Memories are forever stored and accomplishments continue.

Achievements are not stolen: they remain to be found once more.

Memories and accomplishments, personal history, and knowledge just have to be accessed.

That's what we do.

We work to help the person emerge once more. Putting what has been forever stored into use to communicate wishes, needs, feelings, hopes, remembrances, dreams.

We are the cheerleaders who help to build the confidence and inner strength needed to push through the tragedy of injury or illness.

This is what I do.

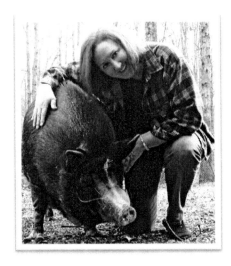

ABOUT LYDIA WINSLOW

A chance viewing of a 1963 television show was the pebble that redirected the flow of Lydia Winslow's life. It was an episode of Dr. Kildare in which Harry Guardino played a man who suffered a stroke and became aphasic. It was then that she returned to school for the degree that would enable her to become a medical speech-language pathologist. She now looks back through forty years of treating individuals with neurological damage, and can still evoke their faces, their names, and each of their unique and challenging situations.

Before becoming a speech pathologist, she worked for MCA Universal writing public relations pamphlets as well as album liner notes. Throughout her various career roles, she continuously wrote, edited, and published civic newsletters. Lydia Winslow's non-fiction work has been published in two internationally recognized hobby periodicals.

She resides in the upstate of South Carolina with her husband, their cat, dog, and famous potbellied pig, Peggy. She continues to work in the field of speech and language pathology, and continues to collect what she calls "favorite patients."

This is Lydia Winslow's first published memoir.